NATIONAL INSTITUTE SOCIAL SERVICES LIBRARY

Volume 37

A PLACE LIKE HOME

A PLACE LIKE HOME

A Hostel for Disturbed Adolescents

W. DAVID WILLS

Routledge
Taylor & Francis Group

LONDON AND NEW YORK

First published in 1970 by George Allen & Unwin Ltd

This edition first published in 2022
by Routledge
4 Park Square, Milton Park, Abingdon, Oxon OX14 4RN
605 Third Avenue, New York, NY 10017

Routledge is an imprint of the Taylor & Francis Group, an informa business

British Library Cataloguing in Publication Data
A catalogue record for this book is available from the British Library

ISBN: 978-1-03-203381-5 (Set)
ISBN: 978-1-00-321681-0 (Set) (ebk)
ISBN: 978-1-03-206718-6 (Volume 37) (hbk)
ISBN: 978-1-03-206734-6 (Volume 37) (pbk)
ISBN: 978-1-00-320359-9 (Volume 37) (ebk)

DOI: 10.4324/9781003203599

Publisher's Note
The publisher has gone to great lengths to ensure the quality of this reprint but points out that some imperfections in the original copies may be apparent.

Disclaimer
The publisher has made every effort to trace copyright holders and would welcome correspondence from those they have been unable to trace.

A PLACE LIKE HOME
A Hostel for Disturbed Adolescents

by

W. David Wills

With a Foreword by
Dame Eileen Younghusband

London
GEORGE ALLEN & UNWIN LTD
RUSKIN HOUSE MUSEUM STREET

FIRST PUBLISHED IN 1970

PRINTED IN GREAT BRITAIN
in 11 on 12 point Fournier
BY T. & A. CONSTABLE LTD
EDINBURGH

TO 'MRS S.'

FOREWORD

by

Dame Eileen Younghusband

The venture described in this book began with a suggestion to the Buttle Trust for Children that valuable experimental work could be done by setting up a hostel for boys leaving schools for maladjusted children who had no settled home and needed a bridge between leaving school and finding for themselves an independent life in the community. The Buttle Trust decided to set up an *ad hoc* exploratory committee. A member, Miss Leila Rendel, then Director of the Caldecott Community, gave the committee much valuable advice about the necessarily high staff/boy ratio, the type of house that would be needed and the importance of keeping numbers small. In 1959 the Buttle Trust decided to go ahead with the project on the general lines suggested by the committee. The Trust asked the National Association for Mental Health to take responsibility for setting up this pioneer hostel and offered a substantial grant for the purpose. The NAMH agreed to this proposal.

Local authorities in the London area were circularized and assured the NAMH that a subsidized fee of £10 per week would not be prohibitive and that the initiative of providing a hostel would be welcome. Once this was certain, the next problem was to find a suitable house and a warden under whom a staff could be recruited. In the event, the warden came before the house because by a rare stroke of good fortune David Wills, who for years had had an international reputation for his work in residential schools for maladjusted children, unexpectedly became available in 1961 and agreed to become warden of a so far non-existent hostel. The Buttle Trust and the NAMH both seized the opportunity. Thus David Wills was employed while the search for a house went forward. This enabled him to share in the decision about the house which was eventually bought, to visit schools from which boys might come, as well as making contact with local authorities and professional colleagues.

The search for a house went on for many frustrating months. In 1961 the NAMH had to report that 198 houses had been considered, 33 of them in detail, and three times a suitable house had been found but planning permission was refused. Finally, in 1962 a suitable house was found in Bromley and, having overcome all the difficulties of planning permission and adaptation of the premises, the hostel finally came into existence in September 1963 with the admission of the first boy. It was named Reynolds House in memory of Mr H. Reynolds, Director of the Buttle Trust, whose sudden death had cast a shadow over the project for which he had worked so tirelessly.

The purchase and equipment costs of Reynolds House were met by the Buttle Trust, which also met deficiencies in running costs for the first five years. Inevitably costs crept steadily higher over the years while at the same time the difficulty of maintaining a steady number of residents also rocked the financial boat. By 1968 the real per capita cost had risen to nearly £25 per week. High costs are, however, an inevitable difficulty in experiments where small numbers of residents and a proportionately large number of skilled staff are of the essence of the experiment.

The NAMH appointed a management committee to support David Wills and his staff and also took responsibility through its headquarters for servicing the management committee, the accountancy work, maintenance of property, the collection of fees, and negotiations with local authorities on financial matters. The Buttle Trust was also closely and actively concerned with developments at Reynolds House. These are a few background facts by way of introduction to David Wills' own vivid account of the project. It is obvious that in much of what he describes he is calling upon his own rich past experience of maladjusted young people as well as his knowledge as a psychiatric social worker. In spite of this sureness of touch and in spite of a strong and united team and an actively interested and helpful psychiatrist and committee of management, it is obvious on almost every page that the work was full of stress for everyone concerned in it, and that only people with much wisdom, skill and compassion could respond appropriately to the residents' demands and remain in control of the situation. This book indeed demonstrates, as other accounts of work with severely damaged and homeless young people have done, that to help them into adulthood and independence is no question of providing ordinary lodgings or hostels; rather it calls for extremely expensive facilities run by skilled staff with many of the attributes of archangels. This book will certainly add greatly to our understanding of the personalities, life experience and needs of maladjusted boys in their 'teens. The lessons to be drawn from it are disturbing in relation both to prevention and treatment. David Wills' account shows vividly the extent of deprivation suffered by such young people and the amount that adults must be able to give them if they are to be set upon a less turbulent course in life.

I have often met such young people during many years in a London juvenile court and can confirm both the penetration of David Wills' assessment as well as having a nostalgic wish that some of those juvenile court boys could have gone to Reynolds House. As a Buttle Trustee I feel proud that the Trust should have shown the far-sighted imagination to start and finance this project and I hope that this book will be read with profit by many of those who are trying in various capacities to help boys and girls who otherwise grow into adulthood permanently handicapped emotionally and socially.

PREFACE

AND ACKNOWLEDGEMENTS

In attempting to give an account of the work upon which my wife and I were engaged during the five years preceding our retirement I have many people to thank.

Chronologically the Buttle Trust come first as they initiated the project and provided the capital. Their interest was much more than financial. The hostel was named after Mr H. Reynolds, a senior officer of the Trust who had seen the work through its preliminaries but unhappily died just as the hostel was opening. They were represented on the Committee of Management by two of their officers, one of whom, Commander G. R. A. Don, R.N., was also involved in all the preliminaries and served with great faithfulness until the Committee was dissolved shortly after my retirement. His help and interest were far beyond the line of duty, and it was a great pleasure to receive visits at one time or another, usually under his guidance, from all the members of the Trust.

The Buttle Trust asked the National Association for Mental Health to accept responsibility for the Hostel, which they accepted. To them I am grateful not only for the opportunity to do an exciting and stimulating piece of work, but also for the unfailing encouragement, support and trust of their officers. Unless he is so insensitive that he ought really to be doing a different job, the most experienced residential worker needs to feel that he has someone to lean on, and the NAMH supplied this need abundantly. During the first three years, until she left the NAMH, my 'contact' was Miss Leonora Elphick, who was responsible for the Association's residential services; but during the whole period, and since, I have been conscious of the friendly interest and energetic support of the Association's General Secretary, Miss Mary Applebey. She spent much tedious time both on this book and on the Report to the Buttle Trust, making numerous valuable suggestions, as also did Miss Morna Smith. I derived much pleasure from this strengthening support, not only because of its intrinsic value, but also because of the friendly and ungrudging spirit in which it was given. The NAMH also provided the Chairman of the Committee of Management, the Hon. Mrs Peter Vanneck. Her frequent visits gave joy to my wife and myself, and great pleasure to the whole community: I still remember the amazed incredulity with which two boys watched her one evening as she worked in the garden in the rain. Her unassuming but informed and enthusiastic interest was a constant source of stimulation.

The resident team was a small one. Apart from successive au pair girls it consisted only of four people, my wife and myself and our respective deputies. I am happy to say that during the greater part of the period they were the same four people, as my wife's deputy Mrs Gertrude Skilton was with us for nearly five years, and Mr Ronald Martin was my deputy for nearly three. Mrs S., as she has been affectionately known for many years to numbers of children, young people and colleagues, was a former colleague and dear friend, but Mr Martin was new both to us and (in a professional sense) to the work. Readers will learn in what follows something of what we owed to them, and I am glad to place on record my deep sense of obligation. Mrs S. shared with my wife what I have described as 'the thick end of the stick', which they both grasped with mature resolution combined with feminine gentleness and sensitivity. With a skill and patience at which I never cease to wonder they kept all the domestic arrangements on a steady even keel, but still had energy and somehow found the time for a highly skilled, meaningful and fruitful relationship with the boys, whose demands on them, practical and emotional, were unceasing.

By our visiting part-time staff we were also remarkably well-served but I am sure I shall not be misunderstood if I single out the three who were with us longest: Dr Doreen Sherwood-Jones, the psychiatrist, Mrs Pamela Ingram, the secretary who was so much more than that, and Mr Iain Campbell, who has been given the undignified and totally inadequate title of 'spare man'. I have praised them in what follows; I give them now my warmest thanks.

Our work was the team-work of a central resident team, and a larger team which included the visiting staff, the NAMH and the Committee; any success we had was a combined success, and not mine alone. And perhaps I may also give my thanks to the anonymous editor from the National Institute for Social Work Training, who, among many other felicitous textual amendments, substituted the plural first person for the intrusive and egotistical singular of which I had been too often guilty. The work was the work of us all and the responsibility of us all. But what appears between these pages is my responsibility alone. I have received much help from many sources and I wish I had produced something more worthy of it; but that egotism which the editor saw fit to admonish has led me to reject some at least of the counsel that has been offered. The work was ours; but for any theory, opinion or interpretation that appears between these covers, I alone must take the blame.

D. W.

CONTENTS

———

CHAPTER ONE

A BOY WITH A PROBLEM

When Thomas was still an infant he had a serious internal disorder and had to go to hospital. There was some doubt whether he would live, and he was in hospital for several months. He was no stranger to hospitals – there had been complications when he was born, and he had remained for some months after his mother went home. This time, however, a different kind of complication emerged, one that was to have a profound effect on his whole life. When Tommy eventually returned home, fully recovered, he found that he had been supplanted – there was a new baby who occupied his mother's time and attention and Tommy resented it. In this he behaved like millions of other infants when another baby comes along, but in Tommy's case the trouble was exacerbated by the fact that he had been wrenched – by illness – from his mother, without that process of emotional weaning by which the child learns first that he and his mother are separate beings, and second that although they are separate, the mother's love and care are all-embracing and absolutely to be relied on.

Tommy was spiteful to John, slapped him, tried to steal his little bits of infantile property, expressing his resentment without inhibition in every way that is open to a two-year-old. Just as millions of babies resent the intrusion of a newcomer in the family, so millions of mothers cope successfully with the situation, assuring the 'supplanted' child of their continuing love and care, often with such success that the older child comes to identify with the mother and to share in some measure her attitude to the new baby. Not so Tommy's mother. For whatever reason, she was quite unable to understand or to cope with his distress and jealousy. In a very short time Tommy's fear had become a tragic reality. He *was* supplanted. His mother had reacted not with understanding and love but with harshness and punishment until Tommy felt himself – rightly – to be totally rejected. His young life became a kind of quest to fill the vaguely apprehended void which the withdrawal of his mother's love had left: by the acquisition of material objects, often belonging to his mother; by wandering off in search of he knew not what; by war against his supplanter and against the mother who had disappointed him, and against all whom she loved.

He became depressed and sought to defend himself against his depression by various kinds of bizarre behaviour and by aggressiveness. In short, he became a very disturbed and difficult child indeed, but to his mother an uncontrollably 'naughty' one.

By the time Tommy was five he had been referred to the child guidance clinic. The clinic early discovered that there was little they could do with mother or child so long as they remained together fanning the fires of each other's animosity, so they arranged for Tommy to go to a boarding school for maladjusted children. It was hoped that when the sore spot was removed it might be possible to do something to mitigate the mother's deeply felt resentment against her son, and that perhaps after a few terms it might be possible for him to return home. In this they were disappointed; failure was so complete that it became impossible for Tommy even to spend his holidays at home, and every time a holiday came round some fresh arrangement had to be made. From time to time another home visit was tried, but always with the same result; Tommy and his mother remained like tinder and spark that could not be brought near one another without fear of conflagration. Tommy would 'torment' his brothers and sisters, defy his mother and father, react to rebuke with violent aggressiveness, and was generally 'impossible'.

Meanwhile, at school, he was relatively happy. True, he transferred his sibling jealousy to his schoolfellows, especially the younger ones, perpetually tormenting and annoying them. True, he transferred to the staff of the school his disgust and hatred of his parents. These adults, however, knew that Tommy was not a wicked child but a desperately unhappy one. To all his exasperating symptoms they responded with understanding, with sympathy, with love. Tommy had been fortunate in being sent to an exceptionally good school – for schools for maladjusted children vary in quality like any other schools – like indeed all human institutions; and he made a very good, warm relationship with the headmaster and his wife. They, familiar with Tommy's background and history, believed it to be their duty so far as humanly possible to provide the unswerving, unconditional affection his mother had been unable to provide and to check him, when his symptoms displayed themselves, with consistent firmness but without harshness or animosity (perhaps that is what George Lyward means when he talks about 'stern love'), assuring him always that however he might misconduct himself and however they might find it necessary to rebuke him, their love was always there, and was entirely unaffected by what he might do.

Slowly Tommy responded, but progress was very slow indeed; it is difficult for someone else to take the place of a rejecting mother because after all it is not merely love the child is seeking, but *her* love, and it is probably true to say that no-one else can ever be a real substitute. But Mr and Mrs Penfold[1] persevered, and Tommy did improve, was somewhat less unbearable to other children, and began to find it possible to place *some* trust in adults, so that by the time he reached school-leaving age he was, while still a nuisance, no longer an unmitigated, insufferable nuisance.

Towards the end of his school life he went home for a holiday. It was an abysmal failure. When he mildly teased his brothers and sisters (mildly that is, for Tommy) his mother reacted with unbridled and unconcealed animosity. We are not – let it never be forgotten – to blame her for this; she was reacting instinctively – as was Tommy – to the circumstances in which she found herself, and defending, to the best of her ability, her young against attack, as any mother will and should. But she had alas, become incapable of sympathetic understanding so far as Tommy was concerned and, however much she tried, was incapable of simulating a love she did not feel. All this of course simply exacerbated Tommy's troubles, and everyone was unfeignedly thankful when the holiday ended.

There remained only one more term before Tommy's school life was due to end. What was to be done with him? 'We cannot have him home,' said his distracted father. 'I've been married over twenty years now, and my wife says that if *he* comes here, *she* will go somewhere else. I know she will. I can't have my marriage breaking up after all these years, all because of one of my six children.' It was clear indeed that even if Tommy's mother had not refused to have him, it would have been fatal for him to return home, and here perhaps she displayed more wisdom than she knew, or was credited with. In a few months all his old trouble would have returned. He would have become what the psychiatrists call a 'depressive', and before long would have found his way to a psychiatric hospital. It was clear that his emotional state was still so uncertain that probably any warden of an ordinary working boys' hostel would have found him too difficult to handle and similar consequences might well have ensued. Any ordinary foster mother, or any 'good motherly soul' taking in lodgers would equally have found him impossible. Where *was* he to go?

In the event Tommy was lucky. His headmaster had heard that the

---

[1] I have given 'Mr and Mrs Penfold' a pseudonym to make sure that 'Tommy' cannot be identified.

National Association for Mental Health was about to start a hostel for just such boys as Tommy, of whom there are very many. For his story is unique only in the sense that every human story is unique. In the sense that he was an unhappy, emotionally disturbed youth due to leave a special boarding school, but with no adequate home to receive him, and needing skilled care and attention until he reached maturity, he was by no means alone. How many there are it is impossible to say. When I was in charge of a school for maladjusted children I was constantly being perplexed and distressed by this very problem. When, therefore, the NAMH, asked me if I would like to take charge of their proposed hostel, I was very happy to spend the last five years of my working life helping those who, like myself, had recently left a school for maladjusted children.

CHAPTER TWO

– AND A PLACE FOR HIM TO GO

The hostel was called Reynolds House and accommodated twelve boys. This number was not hit upon just by chance. Our hope was that the staff might supplement the generally ameliorative influence of the hostel environment in two principal but very important ways: through personal one-to-one relationships between staff and boys on the one hand, and through the use of group dynamics on the other. To be successful with the former, small numbers were essential, as the kind of relationship aimed at was of the family type, and indeed it was hoped that at one level the community would live and operate very much as a family. For this kind of approach and relationship it was hardly practicable to try to cope with more than twelve at the most, and eight might have been ideal, though in the early stages of planning the proposal to restrict accommodation to eight was rejected. It was rejected because the other aspect of community life that was envisaged – the use of group influences or group dynamics through the medium of shared responsibility was hardly feasible with so small a number. For this purpose twenty-four or thirty might have been ideal, and the smallest practicable number was twelve. Twelve therefore as the maximum from one point of view and the minimum from the other, seemed to be the optimum, so twelve was the number decided upon. Experience brought no modification of our view on this subject, and did strongly confirm the view that twelve was something like a minimum for the satisfactory exercise of shared responsibility. During the rather long building-up period, when numbers were less than twelve, this aspect of the work was almost a total failure, but once twelve was reached it became a great success. The sceptic may be tempted to say 'Naturally, you didn't expect it to succeed with less than twelve, so you didn't put into it what was necessary to make it succeed.' He will be mistaken. I entirely forgot I had said that twelve was the fewest with which shared responsibility could be successful, and as I have always used this instrument I put it into operation as soon as the hostel opened. As the months went by I became more and more depressed at its failure and eventually expressed the opinion that shared responsibility was a splendid thing for full-time residential establishments but was not suitable for hostels, giving reasons. I had no sooner done so than things began to improve, the house-meeting becoming dynamic and purposeful, and this change came about as soon as the numbers reached twelve.

This early period was a difficult one in other respects. During the first twelve months there were no fewer than seven 'non-stayers', two of them being expulsions. I would have been prepared to expel them all and start again if necessary, but happily it was not. I expelled the two after due warning, for deliberate, cold-blooded and repeated violence against their fellows. There was at that time no other way of dealing with them, but by the middle of the following year a sufficient body of public opinion, and the means for expressing it, had been built up to make such an action never again necessary. But if drastic action had not been taken in the first year, such free expression of public opinion might never have been established. The other five transients in the first year went for a variety of reasons, which are discussed in Chapter Nine. But during the ensuing four years there were only three such transients, and one of them was clearly connected with the impending retirement of three of the senior staff. The staff envisaged by the NAMH was a warden and matron and a deputy for each, a part-time psychiatric social worker and a psychiatrist on a sessional basis (one session a fortnight) plus part-time cleaners and cooks. In the event, because I am by training a psychiatric social worker and therefore carried the dual role, a part-time secretary was appointed instead. I am not putting this forward as an ideal arrangement in all circumstances, but it suited us very well and worked out happily in practice. The post of social worker in residential establishments other than hospitals is a very new one, and the role has yet to be formulated with any clarity and precision. Even when the social worker has a perfectly clear idea of his (or, of course, and more probably, her) function, this has still to be accepted by the residential worker, who at present rarely understands it fully and tends to resist it as threatening to his own role and status. While of course the social worker must know and be known by the residents, I see her as working primarily not with them but with their families. I see her as carrying out a two-way interpretive role between family and child and between family and residential worker. She should not be involved, unless very exceptionally, in interpreting residential worker to child, because too many susceptibilities are involved though she may have a very useful function in the opposite direction. Her own direct work with the child begins when he resumes normal life outside the institution, though for

reasons I shall give in discussing aftercare (Chapter Nine) I believe
the residential worker also has a place here.

The head of an institution who has maintained some kind of contact
with families does not always realize how much there is to do nor how
much more effectively this can be done by a trained social worker, and
is apt to resent what he sees as interference, and feels as a threat to his
lordly authority as head. The social worker on the other hand has
rarely had any real experience of residential work with all its stress and
tension, and can easily present herself as an officious busybody who
hardly knows the elementary facts of residential life. There is much
careful and patient work to be done before a happy working relationship can be established, both in general as between the two professions
and in particular when a social worker takes up her post. By virtue
of the skills in which she has been trained, the onus of creating a good
relationship rests at present more heavily upon the social worker than
on her residential colleague.

We did not resolve any of these problems at Reynolds House; we
simply avoided them by making use of the fact that I was technically
qualified to do either, and I did both. The difficulties involved in my
attempting, as social worker, to act in an interpretive way between a
family and myself as residential worker, arose but rarely because in so
many cases the breach between the boy and his family had already
been found to be final and irremediable before he came to us. That was
in fact in very many cases the reason for his coming to us.

It was assumed that the Warden and Matron would be a married
couple, and while other arrangements can doubtless work successfully,
a married couple has many advantages. The boys tend to adopt a more
or less filial attitude to the senior man and woman and this is on the
whole desirable – it is in any event inevitable with young people who
are to all intents and purposes otherwise parentless. Such a relationship
is more realistic and more easily sustained where its subjects are man
and wife. Again, close and indeed intimate co-operation is essential
between Warden and Matron and this is obviously much easier for a
married couple. Finally, and this is perhaps the most important point,
it is of the utmost value to present to the residents a living example of
a successful matrimonial relationship. Most of the residents, as we
have seen, had no experience of ordinary happy family life, and
were apt to be cynical about the married state, and to have a
regrettably primitive and contemptuous attitude to the other sex.
The presence therefore in a central position of a couple whose successful marriage is manifestly based on mutual affection and respect,

can do much to mitigate the deplorable effects of earlier, unhappy experiences.

In our kind of set-up at Reynolds House, it was the women who had the rough end of the stick. The role they adopted, as much from force of circumstances than from conscious policy, was one that is tending to be regarded as old-fashioned and unprofessional. It was certainly very strenuous. As the status of residential child-care workers rises, there is an increasing tendency for the trained-woman to be regarded as someone who is not directly concerned with domestic duties. I am among those who ardently advocate the raising of the status of the residential worker, but this attitude has its dangers. Status does not depend on what work a person does, but rather upon the value that society places upon that work. The value of the housewife and mother in our society can hardly be over-estimated, and if such women are uneasy about their status, that is partly at least because we still carry over, in our attitude to them something of the Victorian contempt for the domestic worker. So far as the professional housemother is concerned (and I much prefer this term to 'Matron', with its overtones of starchy hospital discipline) so far as *she* is concerned, I am sure there is a value in her being still concerned with domestic affairs, though not overwhelmed by them, and the much desired rise in her status must be brought about – in part at least – by a change in our attitude to domestic chores.

In the early days of training for residential child care I used to be critical of the courses because they seemed to be largely devoted to the business of domestic arrangements and a superficial introduction to various kinds of craft work. I have been happy to see over the years (and especially recently) an increasing emphasis on the dynamics of human growth and behaviour and even on group dynamics. This is all to the good, but it will be a great pity if in our new professionalism we forget that residential work is in a real sense domestic and that even if we do not strive to be parent substitutes we are nevertheless invested by the children with parental roles. One of the skills of the worker is to make constructive use of the role in which the child sees him, and the worker-child relationship is more difficult to establish if we do not fill the expected role in a familiar way. All this means that our trained professional worker must be prepared to be involved to some degree with household chores and of course this applies more to the women than to the men, though not exclusively to them. There is another point in this context that is sometimes not understood by young workers, who are heard to say 'I don't have time to make relationships with the children.' Effective relationships do not exist in a vacuum, but arise out of and complement a practical contact, without which it is extremely difficult if not impossible to establish them. That practical contact might be mending a boy's shirt for him or helping him to mend his motor bike, washing up with him or playing Monopoly. The pity is that the women's points of contact are often so much more boring than the men's, and the problem is to effect a proper balance between the necessary household affairs, and opportunities for more relaxed and interesting contacts.

We never found a satisfactory solution to this problem at Reynolds House, and that is why I say the women had the rough end of the stick. They sometimes felt almost overwhelmed by their domestic responsibilities; or rather not so much overwhelmed by *them*, as by the fact that they carried a large burden of additional demands made by the residents, demands which, I strongly suspect, would have been fewer and less insistent if their mother-role had not been reinforced by the fact of their being obviously engaged in traditional mother-functions. I suspect that it was easier for the boys to talk confidentially to a woman in an apron, engaged in ironing, than to someone with nothing else to do but to listen to them.

One of the two women staff members was on duty every evening (as well as for part of the day) so as to be 'around' when the boys were in the house. For better or worse, the evening was spent largely in the kitchen or the laundry, or sewing in the quiet room, so that the amount of time available for relaxed association with the residents was very small indeed. But, as I have just said, this familiar domestic role was one which was more comprehensible and acceptable to the residents than that of the 'professional', and made the women, in spite of their domestic preoccupations, more easily approachable. Indeed it was very much easier for a resident to have a casual but private conversation with a woman than with a man, because a boy who wanted to talk privately with me, for example, had first to separate me from the other residents, whereas he could often find a woman alone in the kitchen or laundry, and could start talking to her without the daunting preliminary of saying 'Can I have a talk with you in private?' For this reason, as well as by reason of their mother-relationship, the women tended much more than the men to be the repositories of the boys' confidences. Very often when a boy wanted to convey something to me, something that he was proposing to do, or some problem that was worrying him, he would begin by confiding in my wife or her deputy in the perfect confidence that it would be passed on to me. By this means the responsibility for providing an opportunity for private conversation was passed on to me with no direct word spoken.

All this was admirable and excellent, but very exhausting for the women concerned, and it was very fortunate that during most of the five years I had the co-operation and support of two such devoted, skilled and gifted women, both of whom were prepared to combine a 'humble' domestic role with that of a professional social worker in a residential setting.

The same good fortune attended the selection of non-resident domestic staff, the cooks and cleaners. These were usually four or five in number, each doing a few hours a day, but not all on the same days. They provided each week forty hours of cleaning time and twenty-four hours of cooking. None of them came on Sundays, when the whole of the domestic work had to be done between us, and on weekdays only the evening meal was cooked by the visiting staff.

These women formed a fine and loyal team of colleagues who not only carried out their primary function with good will and competence, but also took a real and valuable interest in the whole work of the hostel. Some of them were women of exceptionally high calibre, and we were able to call upon them as occasional evening 'reliefs' when my wife or the deputy matron was on holiday, together with the excellent and admirable secretary who served the hostel during most of the five years. Although, technically, she only worked at the hostel fifteen hours a week, and although she had her own home to run and her own family to look after, the contribution that she made can hardly be measured.

During most of the five years we enjoyed the services of what we called, officially, a resident domestic, but who in practice was very much more than that. She was usually a Swiss girl who came for six to twelve months on a modified au pair basis while she was improving her English. In this way we were admirably served by a series of exceptionally charming young women. They were girls of some education with professional aspirations, and it was very useful to have in the house a personable young woman who, while young and attractive enough to appeal to the boys, could at the same time present to them an acceptable standard of feminine conduct.

Among this welter of women there were also men: myself, my deputy, and a 'spare man' who came in one evening a week. The office of deputy in such hostels is not an easy one to carry out. The man concerned must on the one hand adapt himself to the authority, ideas and methods of the warden, but must at the same time have a sufficiently strong and independent personality to be able to exercise authority on his own behalf in the warden's absence. The man who can do both with equal success is rare, and the more successful he is in one of these roles, the less successful he is likely to be in the other. There is a chronic shortage of good men in residential work, so one cannot expect to keep a good deputy very long.

The first deputy-warden, whose wife was deputy matron, left after a year to take a Home Office course which was offered to him a year sooner than he expected. They are now in charge of a hostel for maladjusted children. The second, a trained teacher from the dominions, stayed only two or three weeks and left without notice after a bloody affray with one of the residents. The third also left after a year to take further training, but the fourth we had with us, I am happy to say, for the remainder of the five years. He was an older man, in his forties, without training or relevant professional experience who had decided, at some financial sacrifice, to take up residential work with under-privileged young people, from idealistic motives. There were about three months with no deputy at all, during which the presence of the 'spare man' proved to be an enormous boon.

One of the chronic problems of the small hostel is that of providing for relief during time off, and particularly during holidays as the staff is necessarily so small that it is difficult for them to 'cover' for each other. However few the number of residents, there are still twenty-four hours in each day and seven days in each week, and the staff therefore cannot be reduced in proportion to the numbers of the residents. Many hostels of the size of Reynolds House are staffed with only one man, so that every minute of free time he enjoys is dependent on someone coming in from outside. This is not to imply that his women colleagues are necessarily incapable of handling adolescent boys, even when they present the additional hazard of being maladjusted; but women in a residential establishment, and certainly women at Reynolds House, tend always to be so occupied with their own function and role that they could hardly do the work of absent men without serious risk of being overburdened. It must further be said that few responsible committees of management would be happy with a situation in which a woman was for frequent and long periods in sole charge of a group of young men whose very presence in the establishment was due to the fact that *some* of them are prone, to a greater or lesser degree, to acts of violence. For these reasons the NAMH thought it imperative that there should be two full-time men on the staff. It was recognized that the social work aspects of the job did not provide full-time occupation for two men, so they must be (and were) willing to help with domestic chores and accept responsibility for the 'handymanning'. In fact, throughout the five years, tradesmen were called in for repair or maintenance jobs only for really major repairs or those calling for a high degree of technical expertise.

Even so, unless one man were to be on duty twenty-four hours a day for weeks on end while the other was on leave, further help was necessary. Most of the boys were out at work all day, but the occasions when there was no boy in the house were extremely rare. In addition to the odd unemployed boy, there are the vagaries of the shift system, and of free half days and days off, and as long as there was even one boy about the place it was not possible really to relax. So we needed relief at holiday times, but in a regime such as the one at Reynolds House, where social order depended more on a good relationship than on the imposition of authority, it was essential that any person relieving in this way should be familiar with the boys, and have some sort of relationship, however superficial, with each one of them. It was pointless therefore merely to call upon the 'spare man' when one of us was on holiday, so we looked for someone who would come in one evening every week. That weekly evening would enable him to get to know the boys and to keep in touch with what was happening at the hostel, so that he was equipped to operate from a secure base when he was called upon during holiday times to come in a little oftener. This arrangement had the further advantage that it enabled all the resident staff to attend the case conference which was held fortnightly on the evening that the 'spare man' was on duty.

I imagined we should have great difficulty in finding a man to fill this bill, but we picked a winner straight away. He served in this capacity the whole time (and still does), and I will not attempt to describe his skills and virtues because they would sound too good to be true. The fact that he served all those years in this very difficult capacity is tribute enough, and he earned the admiration and affection of everybody connected with the place, from the Chairman of the Management Committee, to the newest five-hours-a-week cleaning woman, including, of course, all the residents.

It remains only to refer to one other staff member, the visiting psychiatrist, who reluctantly and to our great regret resigned her appointment after four years because of increasing domestic responsibilities. The psychiatrist, who gave one session a fortnight, was vital and indeed integral to our work. She primarily had an advisory and supportive role in relation to the staff. Her customary duties were:

1 to help in the selection of residents,

2 to attend the fortnightly case conference,

3 to interview, when occasion demanded, the odd resident at the request of the case conference (or at his own request) to diagnose, advise or encourage; obviously there was not enough time for her to carry out actual psychotherapy.

In addition to the foregoing, she was always willing to talk on the telephone, to me or, in my absence, my deputy, if any difficult situation arose; to suggest, advise, or merely to sympathize – and that is a valuable service! And of course she maintained such liaison as was necessary with any medical authorities or persons concerned with the residents.

Her normal procedure at her fortnightly visits was first to join the family at its evening meal, which gave her the opportunity at least to be able to identify the residents by name, and as time went on to get to know them. If a prospective resident was visiting with a view to being accepted, he would be seated near her so that she could form an impression of him in an entirely informal way. Because it was our aim to discourage the residents from thinking of themselves as in any way abnormal, her psychiatric role was as far as possible soft-pedalled. On the odd occasion when it was not possible to hold a formal case conference owing to the absence of staff members on holiday, she would still visit, discussing briefly with whoever was in charge any problems that might have arisen, and spend the rest of the evening fraternising with the residents, which might include a game of Monopoly or Scrabble, or even helping with the dishwashing. It is a tribute to her skill as a psychiatrist, her friendliness as a person and her charm as a woman, that several of these adolescent boys from time to time sought her help and guidance. Her successor, a man, was able to slip readily and easily into the same kind of happy relationship that she had established.

Every alternate Monday evening then, the resident staff foregathered after dinner in our flat with the psychiatrist and a social worker from the NAMH, while the 'spare man', with notable competence, held the fort below stairs. We had a pleasant, rambling, informal chat and although there was both plan and structure, we made sure they were our servants, not our masters.

The agenda might have up to four sections. The first part contained the names of boys being considered for admission, the second contained the names of three residents whom it was proposed to discuss, and who came up seriatim in alphabetical order, though any boy might be brought forward who was undergoing some crisis or emergency; the third contained the names of any boys being considered for discharge; and the fourth contained the names of any ex-residents whom it was thought proper or expedient to discuss. As often as not the agenda contained only the matter of current residents and only very rarely would there be four parts.

Apart from discussing and deciding upon admissions and discharges, the main functions of the Monday discussions were to act as a clearing house for information about residents, and ideas and suggestions for their treatment; and to provide a medium through which the advice and support of the psychiatrist could be made available to the staff.

In order that the non-resident members (i.e. the psychiatrist and the NAMH social worker) might be kept abreast of developments, I made periodic progress notes on each resident, which were distributed as soon as they were written, usually the week before the boy in question was due to be discussed. In the same way, the non-resident members received copies of all application forms and documents, and of the half-yearly reports that I sent to the authorities sponsoring the boys. Occasionally there would also be present at the conference a child care officer or other social worker specially concerned with one of the boys under review.

Discussion was easy and informal and allowed to wander. This may have taken a longer time but all manner of points were picked up, and perhaps interpreted by the psychiatrist, which in a more formal discussion might well have been missed. We usually finished the names on the agenda in time to have a quick run through the others, or anything else that was of moment or of interest.

The conference was an essential and integral part of the life of the hostel even though the boys knew little of its existence, and I took it so much for granted that I had to be reminded by my colleagues, especially the resident women, whose preoccupation with domestic affairs tended to separate them from the day-to-day therapeutic aspects of the work, that to them it was a necessary and constant source of enlightenment and invigoration, as well as the only opportunity they had for a measured and relaxed consideration of the problems with which they were concerned. It was also almost the only opportunity the rest of us had to hear in a relaxed and unhurried way the valuable contribution the women staff members had to make to the solution of those problems.

We were well served also in the matter of premises. The house took a long time to find, the search extending over more than two years. By 1961 about 200 houses had been examined, 33 of them in detail. In three cases we were denied a suitable house by the refusal of planning permission. Finally in 1962 a suitable house was found in Bromley for which planning consent was readily given. Even so, extensive alterations and additions had to be made, but the end result was highly satisfactory and we were ready to open by the autumn of 1963.

A large and a somewhat smaller room at the front were designated respectively the common room (containing the television set) and quiet room. The term, quiet room, did not mean that a library kind of silence was insisted upon, indeed there was often much rollicking noise there, but merely that in that room radios and record players were banned. It was regarded as absolutely essential that one room should be free of canned music, otherwise verbal contact in a houseful of young people becomes impossible. Our aim was to make this room the focus and centre of the family life, and in this we met with a good deal of success, even though, if a good TV programme was to be seen in the other room, the quiet room might be empty for hours on end. It was used for games, for tea-drinking and chat, for housemeetings and entertaining visitors, that is for all the purposes to which the living room is usually put.

Behind the common room was a fairly spacious dining room with a large window overlooking the big lawn and garden. Built on at the back was the modern kitchen with a laundry to the rear. We also built behind the garage a small workshop which proved, as had been hoped, a great boon. It was equipped at the beginning with a variety of woodwork tools and a bench, but a few months' experience indicated that automechanics' and metal work tools were in greater demand. These were in due course provided, largely by the residents from their own house-meeting funds. The cycle shed proved to be quite inadequate as the residents tended to acquire not only bicycles but also motor cycles and even cars.

There were two floors upstairs, each with four main, one small and one tiny room and the usual offices. The front rooms on each floor were given over to staff accommodation. We did not have the morning sun, but neither did we have boys hanging out of windows to whistle at passing girls. Each of the four back rooms, overlooking the garden, accommodated three residents. The small room on the first floor was the office, and the one above it a guest room.

The furnishing was comfortable and modern. We had taken considerable pains with it, for the aim was that furnishings, curtains and decor in general should reflect good taste according to contemporary standards without being ephemeral in style. A number of pictures were hung, most of them modern lithographs by Barnet Freedman, Edward Bawden, etc. or reproductions of impressionist or post-impressionist painters. In addition, it was later possible, owing to a gift, to ring the changes from a large stock of small reproductions of masters of all periods and styles. At one period the housemeeting decided that they were sick of our 'crummy' pictures, and decided to buy some different ones themselves. They then bought reproductions of paintings by Constable and Turner. Radio, TV and a record player were provided, and there was a small collection of books in the quiet room. The bedrooms contained washbasins and shaver plugs, and a chest of drawers and wardrobe for each resident. Across at least one wall of each bedroom was a large pin-up board. The general feeling of the staff was that it might have been an advantage to have two or three single rooms, but the general structure of the house made this impossible. While it is very nice to have a room of one's own, the wish to have this was sometimes the only factor that inclined a boy to leave the hostel, and if someone was comfortably settled in a private room it might more often have been necessary to bring a little pressure to bear upon those whose continued use of the hostel could no longer be justified.

The criticism was sometimes made by visitors that the standard of living was higher than the boys were accustomed to or could expect to achieve after they had left. This criticism was based partly on the assumption that because much care had been taken in the furnishing and equipping of the place, a disproportionate amount of money had also been spent, but of course that is a very common fallacy. It is true that we used capital to minimize current expenditure, for example, stainless steel jugs and teapots, besides looking very nice, do not have to be replaced as often as earthenware ones, and the comfortably upholstered easy chairs had strong metal frames which cost more but lasted longer than wooden ones. It is true that with central heating throughout, unlimited hot water and free laundry, the boys were getting more for their money than they could expect in the normal course of events, but there are several answers to this criticism, namely:

1 Living standards for all are rising, and the standards provided at Reynolds House were not beyond what might be expected by any good working class family of the future. The present-day working man has his car; his son will have central heating too.

2 It is surely desirable on general, educational grounds to set good standards both in amenity and taste.

3 Socially, the residents were a mixed bag, and some of those from very poor backgrounds could reasonably expect to achieve something very much better than they had been accustomed to.

4 The fact that a boy has had a bad start might be regarded as all the greater reason for giving him now a taste of decent civilized living.

CHAPTER THREE

OTHER BOYS WITH THE SAME PROBLEM

Tommy's headmaster was an old friend and former colleague of mine and it was therefore a pleasure, when we heard about Tommy, to visit his school and hear more about him from my friend, and then to talk to the boy.

Tommy was getting on for sixteen. In fact the average age of boys arriving at Reynolds House during the first five years of its existence was exactly sixteen: the youngest was almost fifteen and the eldest almost eighteen. A boy of that age who has been – as Tommy had – in boarding schools for ten years is, unless he is very unusual, looking forward to the end, however happy he has been there. At my own former school the practice had been for children who were about to leave to have supper with the staff, and there was a half-serious tradition that they should make a speech. The speeches were usually very short, and what most of them amounted to (often consisting simply of these very words) was 'I'm glad I came, and now I'm glad I'm going'. That is how it should be, though sometimes the pleasure of leaving was tinctured with some apprehension about how they would get on with their parents on return. But often they were not nearly as apprehensive as the circumstances warranted. Not only were they full of the optimism of youth (and how they needed it!) but they felt they were no longer children, could 'look after themselves' and, if the worst came to the worst even (now that they were, as they conceived, practically grown up), put their parents in their place! At any rate, they felt that at last they were done with the tutelage of teachers and housemothers, there would be no more 'It's time to do this', or 'time to do that'. 'Have you cleaned your teeth? Let me look at your hands. Do you call those shoes polished?' No more regimentation (and there must be a little even in the best of schools). No more go here, go there. No more bed at 8.30 or 9.30. No more supplication for a new pair of shoes and then having to accept a pair in the style approved by some stuffy adult. From now on (they hoped and believed) they would be free men, earning their living, paying their way, pleasing themselves, living their own lives.

We who are older know how far from actuality these adolescent dreams are, or can ever be; and how unhappy the child – especially the maladjusted child – might well be if they *were* true. But when I went to talk to Tommy I went along with this dream of freedom, as I did with every boy I interviewed about coming to Reynolds House. I had my own subtle, not dishonest reasons for this, and in the sequel I was bountifully justified. I told Tommy, and the others, that he was going to be a free man now. I said 'You're not a kid any longer, and we take it for granted that anyone who comes to Reynolds House is old enough to look after himself. He doesn't need to be told when to take a bath and that sort of thing. He can get out of bed in the morning without having to be thrown out. He can earn his living and pay his way, and so on.' As I described it, it was a kind of small hotel they were invited to come to live in, with my wife and myself as hotel keepers. No 'mothering' and 'fathering', that was the very last thing they wanted, or so they thought. 'Shall I be allowed out in the evenings?' some of them pathetically asked, little suspecting, as indeed we at first little suspected, that one of our greatest problems would be to *get* them to go out in the evenings. 'Great heavens, of course,' I would say. 'Haven't I told you you're a kid no longer, you'll be a free man. You'll come and go as you please. We've no use for a mass of rules and regulations. In fact there are only three rules. I'll tell you what they are *now* and if you don't like them, that's the end of the matter.'

I would then go on to tell them that we had one big rule of over-riding importance. Freedom, I would explain, was something we all wanted and all enjoyed, and we were all for it, but one man's freedom depended in large measure on the next man's willingness to respect it, and if I want freedom myself I must allow it to my neighbour. There-fore Rule Number One was 'Don't do anything that interferes with somebody else's freedom'. If everyone observes that, there's no need for all the pettyfogging little rules, and it was because we thought the boys were old enough and had sense enough to understand and respect *that* rule that we at Reynolds House didn't have dozens of others. Two others, however, we did have. Apart from that first great rule, which was our general rule of life upon which the happiness of the community depended, there were also two specific rules that were laid down as a condition of admission. I made no bones about the fact that *I* was laying down these laws because *I* thought they would tend to the general good, though they might not be able to see it. If they didn't like them they'd better not come, because these rules were not open to discussion. One was that residents must be in the house by 10.30 p.m. (11.00 p.m. on Saturdays). As schoolboys that might seem to them quite late enough, but the chances were that after a time they would find it irksome, so they'd better be warned now. It was ten-thirty and no humbug about it. The generations (I told them) had never seen eye to eye on this question, and I felt quite sure that when the boy I was talking to became a parent, he would quarrel with *his* children about it. So I was not going to argue about it. Ten-thirty was the time, and if they didn't like it they could go somewhere else. I would then go on to temper the rule by saying that of course if they had some *reason* for being out late, I should be very happy to waive the rule in a particular case. In fact, the only thing for which I was likely to refuse late leave was mooching about the streets. Coppers, it was well known, have an ineradicable prejudice against teenagers, and would be only too ready to accuse them of loitering with intent or obstructing the footway or insulting behaviour or any other of those vague and ill-defined offences that are part of the armoury of the police in their war against the young.

In the event one other purpose emerged for which we were unwilling to give late leave, and that was to attend a certain discotheque with a very unsavoury reputation. I could not stop boys from going, but I could (in theory at least) stop them from staying there all night. So that was that. They were to be in by ten-thirty unless late leave had been granted. I never told them, but allowed them to discover with the passage of time, that as they grew older, applying for late leave was allowed insensibly to change into merely telling me, as a matter of courtesy, that they were going to be late. And the other specific rule? Residents must attend the weekly Housemeeting. To one or two boys coming from schools which made use of some form of shared responsibility little explanation of the purpose and function of the Housemeeting was necessary. To others I said simply that its purpose was to watch over the implementation of Rule One. None of us was more than human and were all therefore liable to slip up from time to time in our observance of this very sweeping regulation. At the Housemeeting any such breaches could be discussed. This included breaches by staff as well as by residents, for ours was not to be the kind of staff that could never make a mistake, nor ever be taxed with it. Steps could then be taken to avoid similar breaches in the future. This could be done by simply 'airing' the matter, or by making some specific rule or, if the meeting so wished, by imposing some penalty.

All this I explained to Tommy and to the thirty-seven boys who followed him to Reynolds House in the ensuing five years (as well as to a number who did not). I also explained that I was not offering him a place, but only telling him about the hostel in case he wanted to apply for a place, or we wanted to have him. I had already discussed him with my colleagues on the basis of written information supplied by those responsible for him, and if we had not felt that he seemed at least a likely proposition I should not have gone to see him. Having seen him and talked to his headmaster and any other interested parties I would report to my colleagues on the further information gained and impressions formed, and if by then we were pretty certain we ought to have him, we were ready for the next step. The boy would then be invited to spend a few days at the hostel 'to see how he liked it'. This was not normally done unless we had fairly well made up our minds, because we did not want to raise hopes if there were any foreseeable possibility that they might be dashed. Tommy did not have this experience because he was among our first residents, and at the time he was being considered there was no hostel for him to visit. But that was the general procedure. In spite of the hostility commonly displayed to postulants by those already in residence: 'Blimey! '*E*'s not coming 'ere, is 'e?' and 'Cor! 'Ope we're not going to 'ave *that* twit', were among the milder expressions of sibling jealousy: only one boy ever said he did not want to come, thank you. For some reason he had visited without the usual preliminaries, and when we did see him it was clear that he was far too disturbed to be able to fit into our community anyway.

The criteria upon which we based our judgement as to whether or not a boy was suitable were simple. First, he must have been at a school for maladjusted children. That was the function of the hostel, that was the purpose for which the money had been so bountifully provided by the Buttle Trust, and while we interpreted the term school in so liberal a way as to embrace adolescent units and hostels for the maladjusted, we stuck to this except in two instances both of which we afterwards regretted. I believe that social workers concerned with difficult adolescents in and around London came to regard me as a very hard, narrow, unaccommodating sort of man, and one perhaps who was determined to ensure success for his work by accepting only the 'easy' cases. They would ring up and tell me the most heart-rending stories about a boy they wanted to place with us, and when I said 'Is he at a school for maladjusted children?' would reply 'No. Does that matter? He's *very* maladjusted.' But refuse I did, and that very often too when we had vacancies. For if we had filled those vacancies in mid-term, we should have had none when the end of term arrived and boys were leaving school. For while boys might leave the hostel (and thus create vacancies) at any time, they normally left school to fill those vacancies only at term-end (and latterly only twice a year). Such was the demand for places for these strictly ineligible boys that we could have filled every vacancy as soon as it arose, with the result that in a year or so we should have been quite full with boys who had never seen a school for maladjusted children. So, though it was difficult, we stuck to our guns and refused any boy who had not been to a school for maladjusted children.

We insisted, furthermore, that the boy must come *straight* from school, apart perhaps from any holiday he might take between school and hostel. There must be no going home first 'to see how he gets on', no going home and finding that life at home is absolutely insufferable so that all the old troubles return and all the work of the school has to be done again. In this too I daresay we were thought to be narrow and unaccommodating, but we had our very good reasons. Mr Penfold (for example) had suggested that Tom should come to us because he *knew* that there was no future for Tom at home, because he *knew* that to send him home was not only to risk the break-up of an otherwise satisfactory family; it would mean as certainly as any such thing ever can be forecast, that before long Tom would be in need of residential psychiatric help. Even if there were only one Tom in every school (and I wish there were as few as that), that would be enough to fill Reynolds House several times over.

Of course it is the function of the school for maladjusted children to return the child, healed, it is hoped, or at least helped, to the bosom of his family whenever this is feasible. But sometimes it just is not feasible, and restoration to the family, desirable though this is, must never be thought of as a rigid rule for all cases and in all circumstances. In the treatment of maladjusted children, and of young offenders, as well as in the field of child care generally, inestimable harm has been done, in my view, and lives ruined because people have treated this very desirable aim as an absolute 'must' in all cases, as an immutable rule. Sometimes this is because an unimaginative worker knows only how to operate according to the book, sometimes it is because the people responsible have accepted as universally true the common but pernicious apophthegm that a child's own home is always to be preferred to any other placement.

A headmaster can be pretty certain that some children will do well, he may be doubtful about some, but others, fortunately very few, he knows are going to fail if they go home and that it would be not only pointless but wicked to allow them to do so. Reynolds House exists for those boys. When there are enough Reynolds Houses to cope with all those with a 'failure prognosis', then it might be possible to consider taking some who have been home and failed, but, even so, it is very doubtful whether a hostel is the right place for the difficult rescue operation that is then involved.

Our next condition may also have led to some misunderstanding. The boy must, we said, have made some progress towards stability while he was at the school. 'Ah,' some people may say, 'Wills has got his eye on his outcome figures, so only wants the easy ones.' When I come to describe what kind of boys were received at the hostel, the reader will be able to judge for himself whether there is any justification for this charge. In the meantime there is a simple and sufficient reason for this condition; we could not hope to succeed where the school failed.

It is easy for the staff of a school to see when a child is not making progress – and this is liable to happen in the best of schools. What is *not* easy however, what in fact is often incredibly difficult, is to know whether that child is ever going to make any progress in that particular milieu. Consequently every school from time to time retains a child until school-leaving age, in the perpetual but ultimately disappointed hope that one day he will begin to improve. Can a hostel succeed with such a child? My conviction was, and still is, that we should have been criminally stupid to try. Experience has taught me that in work of this kind an essential element of success is to know exactly what it is you are equipped to do, and to refuse resolutely to do anything else. The moment you start doing something outside your predetermined scope the machinery is thrown out of gear, and your success, even with those you set out to deal with, is immediately reduced. The job the hostel can do is different from the job the school can do. The school has almost complete control over every aspect of the child's life (while he is with them), can modify the environment at any point, can select what influences are to be brought to bear during twenty-four hours of every day. Not so the hostel. During all his working day the hostel resident is subjected to influences, some of them baleful, and to stimuli, some of them pernicious, over which the hostel not only has no control, but of which more often than not it has no detailed knowledge. Very often the same also applies to the boy's evenings and weekends. The school, in other words, is geared to do a fairly intensive therapeutic job, but the hostel is not. The function of the school is to rescue the (emotionally) drowning child and bring him to the point where his nose is above water; the function of the hostel is to place a finger under his nose and keep it there while he practises his strokes, until he is able to swim by himself.

This does not mean that we took (as more than one disappointed sponsor suggested) only the 'cured' cases. If one can talk about a maladjusted child being cured at all, that cure cannot be said to be effective before he has passed through adolescence. We are all maladjusted when we are adolescent, and the adolescent's normal lack of adjustment is apt to be highly exacerbated if he was maladjusted to begin with. Boys are not 'cured' when they come to Reynolds House; on the contrary they are all boys whose relapse and failure can be predicted with a fair amount of confidence unless they can pass from the school into an environment in which they can be sure of skilled and sympathetic guidance and support. But they must show evidence of being able to respond to such skilled care, and those who have not responded to skilled care at the school are not therefore accepted.

The boys who have not responded to the ministrations of the school are a serious problem to which far too little attention so far has been given; but they are not the problem that Reynolds House was established to deal with.

To sum up, the boy must

Firstly, have been at a school for maladjusted children.
Secondly, he must have come straight from that school.
Thirdly, he must have made some positive response to the treatment provided at the school; not 'cured', but showing evidence of being 'curable'.

These three conditions eliminated the need for certain others that might seem necessary or useful. Age, for example, is taken care of by the fact that they came straight from school, and as they are coming to a working boys' hostel they must obviously have reached school-leaving age. Intelligence is covered by the fact that schools for maladjusted children do not normally take boys of very low intelligence. We were never asked to take boys from those few schools which cater only for boys within the grammar school range of ability. Boys with a degree of disturbance so deep or so intractable that they could not be expected to be able to withstand the pressures of normal living, even with the support of Reynolds House, were excluded by our condition about having made some progress towards stability while at school.

To look a little more closely at what boys satisfied these criteria and eventually turned up at Reynolds House: Tommy's case I have described in some detail, and while he is typical in the sense that his need for such a place was absolute, he differed from his fellows, as they differed from each other, in the various ways that human beings do differ from one another. For example, Tom had parents, a home, a family, whereas Chris had (to all intents and purposes) none of these. He was the seventh of eight children of a 'common law marriage'. Shortly after the eighth child was born (Chris being twelve months old) his father disappeared, and his mother, like Sir Albertus Moreton's wife:

> . . . for a little tri'd
> To live without him; lik'd it not, and . . .

disappeared herself, first taking the precaution of placing all her eight children in the care of the local children's department. After a short spell in a residential nursery Chris was fostered, but he was such a fractious, ill-tempered, defiant and unhappy child that the foster-parents could not cope with him, and he was placed at the age of six in a special residential school for maladjusted children. There he remained for ten years, when he came to Reynolds House. The school during all that time had been his only home, the school staff his effective parents, the child care officer virtually his only contact with the outside world. By the time he came to the hostel he had made enormous progress from the apparently ineducable child who had been admitted to the school, but was easily led, and was still at the stage where one does what is right not because it *is* right, but in order to please some loved or admired figure, in his case two members of the school staff. His need was therefore in one sense identical with Tommy's but the circumstances leading up to it were quite different, as were the circumstances of every boy who came to the hostel.

Thirty-eight such boys were admitted during the first five years. Their ages on admission ranged between fourteen years eleven months, and seventeen years ten months, the average being almost exactly sixteen years. Their intelligence was slightly above the middle of the normal range. Their intelligence quotients ranged between 81 and 131, but it can safely be assumed that many of these were under-estimates, especially those in the lower reaches. Our information about I.Q.'s generally dated from the time the boys had first been 'ascertained' as maladjusted, years ago. I do not know whether some I.Q.'s had increased in the meantime, but at the time the tests were made the boys were, so to speak, at the peak of their maladjustment and in many cases therefore would not be functioning up to the standard of which they were capable. Of course we could have had them all re-tested

while they were with us, but this would not have been in keeping with
our general attitude. The line we took with the residents was that,
apart from the fact of not being able to live in the usual way with
parents and their own family, they were perfectly normal people, living
a normal life, and Reynolds House was not some special kind of place
for a special type of person, but a place for them to live because the
normal place, their own home, was not available, or was non-existent.
We did all within our power to discourage them from thinking of
themselves as 'maladjusted', or as interesting problems. The suggestion
was, and I am using that word now in the psychological as well as the
idiomatic sense, that their troubles were over, all left behind at school.
Of course this was not factually true, but it was much more likely to
become true than if we had surrounded them with all the paraphernalia
of intelligence tests and psychiatric interviews and all the rest of it.
This is not to say we ignored such problems as they displayed: only
that we did our best to discourage the growth of psychiatric hypo-
chondria. So we did not have them re-tested, but were quite sure that
many of the I.Q.'s on our records were under-estimates. Tommy, for
instance, was said to have an I.Q. of 81. This was palpable nonsense.
Tommy (who is now in his twenties) has had for years a very responsible job which he might conceivably have *got* (though I doubt it)
but which he certainly could never have *kept* with an I.Q. of 81. His
I.Q. is probably about 110. There were several similar instances, but
on the available I.Q.'s the average was 103. As has been said on p. 37,
not all the boys came strictly from special residential boarding schools
for maladjusted children. The actual number in that category was
twenty-seven. Of the remaining eleven, four came from hostels or
homes in which they had been placed because of behaviour difficulties,
whether or not they were technically or specifically 'hostels for maladjusted children'. Two boys came from the same hostel, which was
run by a local authority for children in care who were maladjusted.

   Two boys came from adolescent units attached to psychiatric
hospitals, which for our purposes counted as schools for maladjusted
children, two came from boarding schools, of which there is now quite
a number which, while not specifically for maladjusted children, are
able to accept a limited number of such children whom they run in
with the normal children of the school. Those were all legitimate
admissions of the kind of boy for whom the hostel was established.
The remaining three, strictly speaking, were not, but were accepted
because in the early days the flow of applicants was very sluggish. One
had been to a school for maladjusted children but had had two years

at home since leaving, and one had been in a children's home awaiting a vacancy in such a school which never materialized. Both of these boys were among the 'transients'. The remaining boy had been since infancy in a small children's home where he remained until adolescence, when he became a problem. He had not been regarded as maladjusted (being still an infant) at the time of his placement in the home, which did receive maladjusted children, and we were able to stretch the point here because I had known both the home and the boy for some years, and this exception we did not regret.

The length of time the boys had spent in their various schools or homes varied from six months to twelve years! This is best expressed in a table, with time approximated to the nearest year, except in the case of the first pair who had each been at an adolescent unit for six months.

Six months	.	2 boys	Six years .	.	1 boy
One year	.	1 boy	Seven years	.	1 boy
Two years	.	5 boys	Eight years	.	2 boys
Three years	.	11 boys	Nine years	.	1 boy
Four years	.	6 boys	Ten years .	.	2 boys
Five years	.	5 boys	Twelve years	.	1 boy

Nine of the boys had been at two schools since they were ascertained to be maladjusted, most of them on transfer from a junior to a senior school. I have always regarded this as a most undesirable practice because it disrupts the affective relationships which are a vital element in the residential treatment of maladjusted children, and I cannot resist this opportunity to make at least a token protest against it. Twenty-one had been admitted to their school or hostel from their own homes, though they did not necessarily still have those homes when they reached Reynolds House, and seventeen had been admitted to their schools from foster-homes or children's homes of one kind or another. Twenty-five were in the care of local authority children's departments who were financially responsible for them while they were at the hostel, and two were in the care of voluntary children's societies. The financial responsibility for the remaining eleven rested with the mental health department of various local authorities, except one who was supported by a local education authority.

There is an anomaly here. Although health authorities maintained about a third of the boys at any time, they did nothing but pay the bill. That is to say, they exercised no social work supervision, and in some cases did not even visit the hostel to see whether it was a suitable place for a boy to live in, or for a ratepayer to spend money on. A truly remarkable situation might, and indeed from time to time did arise. If a local authority paid for a boy out of one pocket, child care, the most careful and skilled liaison was maintained by men and women of extremely high calibre in the main skilled, conscientious and compassionate. If, however, the authority paid for the boy from another pocket, health, there was practically no supervision at all. Sometimes the same authority would be paying for two boys at the same time, carefully and skilfully supervising one, and completely neglecting the other. One would have thought that even from the lowest of motives an authority spending £600-£700 a year on a boy would want to keep in fairly close touch with what their money was buying; while from loftier motives one would have thought that a young person whose circumstances were such that he required the services of an establishment like Reynolds House, was equally in need of skilled and continuing social work care, whether or not he happened to be in care. One mental health department refused to continue to support a boy at the hostel because he had been 'misbehaving', and they wanted to transfer him (I.Q. 97) to a mental deficiency hospital. I cannot believe we should have lost this boy if he had been under the supervision of a skilled social worker who would have recognized that the behaviour complained of was a manifestation of the disorder which brought him to us. Apart from this catastrophe (as it proved to be) the principal consequence of this disparity of treatment seems to have been the increased need for after care by the hostel if a boy was not in care.

The first observation to be made about the boys' background is that most of them were to all intents and purposes homeless. Leaving aside the non-stayers to whom I refer in Chapter Four, we find that only seven of the twenty-eight 'stayers' appeared to have a home in which their own father and mother were living together, including one with adoptive parents. Of these seven, however, two had suffered complete and total rejection by their mothers (Tommy was one, the other was the adopted boy); two had parents who quarrelled openly and violently, one couple separated while the boy was at the hostel; one had a psychopathic father and a grossly inadequate, subnormal mother, and one had a psychopathic mother constantly in and out of hospital. This leaves one boy with an apparently normal home, but with a mother-child relationship which from whatever cause was pathological to an extreme degree. So much for those with two parents living together. Of the remaining twenty-one, five were bastards[1] brought up by the local authority; five were in care because their families had totally disintegrated, six were in effect driven from home by the breakdown of a step-child relationship, for example, Norman, whose family situation was so intolerable that he went to the children's department and asked to be received into care; when his application was rejected he deliberately committed petty thefts with the same end in view, and a fit person order was made by a juvenile court. He is one of our greatest successes. The remaining five had lost a parent by death or separation, and the surviving parent's total inability to cope, either with simply running the home, or with the child's emotional disturbance consequent upon the loss of his parent, led to such a breach in the relationship with the surviving parent that it was no longer possible for them to live together.

It will thus be seen not only that the residents were virtually homeless, but that their homelessness had been brought about in circumstances of trauma and stress that were likely to have a permanent effect on their emotional lives. Some of them, as a result of the work of the schools from which they came, had learned to face this unhappy situation, and to some extent to accept the fact that they no longer had any effective family. Where this had happened, our work of rehabilitation was much facilitated. When such recognition and acceptance of the situation had not been achieved, our work was very much more difficult. Certainly if this was not a condition of success, success was greatly facilitated by it. It should also, however, be stressed, to avoid misunderstanding, that this conception of the school's function relates only to that small group of children represented by the kind that need the services of such a place as Reynolds House. For the majority, of course, the aim of the school is the restoration of the child to its family.

It must further be said that by and large, parents tended to be emotionally unstable, feckless, irresponsible, and antisocial. To this there were occasional exceptions, but of the twenty-three boys who were born in wedlock, five parents were known to have been in psychiatric hospitals, and six in prison. Eight boys had parents who, while never committed to institutions, were described by social workers

---

[1] Bastard. I have been rebuked for using this good English word, but I am impenitent. It has become a term of abuse because of the contempt in which those were once held who had the misfortune to be born out of wedlock. We do not change the public attitude to such people merely by using another term, especially when it is a circumlocutory polysyllabic phrase instead of a simple straightforward noun.

or psychiatrists as subnormal, psychopathic, psychotic, neurotic, violent, grossly inadequate or 'undesirable', or a combination of these. Six of the boys had lost a parent by positive desertion (i.e. by just going off and leaving the family) and seven by negative desertion (i.e. placing the child in care or in a school and then ignoring his existence).

Clearly there was very little contact between residents and their parents. Only two boys willingly maintained regular contact, one with an inadequate but well-disposed father, the other with a mother living abroad. Seven parents made more or less regular attempts to maintain contact, evoking little or no response, or a hostile one. This kind of response (or lack of it) was due, often, to the nature of the parents approaches, which totally lacked sympathy or understanding or even common affection, frequently consisting of long nags. One sad young man made repeated but unsuccessful attempts to evoke a loving response from his adoptive mother, but she was unable to regard him with anything but hostily because he had not cured her of the neurotic condition which had been the reason for her adopting a child. If people who reproach adoption societies saw such consequences they would no longer carp at the precautions these societies take. For the other boys there was no regular contact with parents, and in most cases none at all. Home visits were very rare indeed and were often followed by great emotional distress. Five boys, however, maintained contact with siblings, but two positively refused contact with siblings when offered. Four maintained contact with foster-parents.

The general picture then is of restless young men from disturbed, disrupted, and sometimes chaotic backgrounds, virtually homeless, without normal family relationships or feelings, without experiences of a stable and loving home. The great majority were from working class or poverty-line families, though one was the son and another the stepson of professional men, and four others came from white-collar families. Few of the boys themselves had aspirations beyond those of the labouring class, and among them all there was only one boy with an 'O' Level on arrival at the hostel. We cannot be surprised if such young men were disturbed, anti-social, unable to make relationships and lacking in moral standards or moral stamina.

I have considered, and discarded, the possibility of giving some kind of clinical picture of the problems presented, because within the range of disorder with which we were likely to have to deal, descriptions tend to be vague. Psychiatry is by no means an exact science, and I have learned to distrust diagnoses that are given with perfect assurance. Tentative diagnoses on the other hand are of little use for my present purpose of trying to present a picture of the kind of young man that came to us. Furthermore, our boys had usually been seen by more than one psychiatrist, and their diagnoses, whether assured or tentative, did not always agree. Very often some vague expression like 'general personality disorder' was used, which might mean anything or nothing. Psychiatrists do not all use the same terms of reference, the same criteria or the same terminology, and while our own psychiatrist may have made her own assessments in terms of her own criteria, she did not necessarily reveal them in any detail – rightly as I believe. For these reasons, apart from my own inadequacy in this field, I think there is little to be gained by attempting any formal clinical classification.

Symptoms however are another matter. They are specific and recognizable, their increase and diminution observable. In a realistic sense it is the symptom that brings the boy to a school for maladjusted children and hence to Reynolds House. While we recognized and took account of individual differences and needs, our purpose was not so much to provide specific and individualized treatment for each boy as to provide an environment that was conducive to recovery and stabilization, from which the resident could take, unconsciously or deliberately, those elements that were most helpful to him. We were aware of causes, and equally aware of the possibility of change of symptom (which indeed is sometimes the best that can be hoped for) but by and large the symptom was our guide, and the symptom was what we were concerned with. I appreciate that to some this will seem heretical and unprofessional; but I think it is realistic.

There is one common and characteristic symptom of the maladjusted child. It is like a trademark that is tattooed on his emotional body, the singularity without which it is hardly possible to call a child maladjusted, which can be described as the soil in which the other symptoms take root, or the one which over-arches them all; the inability to form affective relationships with ordinary ease; pathological unclubbability. If one pointer to success in rehabilitation is the degree to which their schools had enabled our boys to 'write off' their families, another is the degree to which they had provided an experience of warm human relationships, and, broadly speaking, a school may be said to have been successful to the degree in which a child had learned to 'relate'. Insofar as the school failed in this task, the work of the hostel was that much more difficult. For *then* the process of teaching how to relate (which can only be done through the experience of affective ties) has to be taken on by the hostel, and of course this becomes increasingly difficult as the child becomes older. It would be helpful if we could make a graded objective scale of a boy's capacity to relate, and I have not the slightest doubt that there are tests known to psychologists by which this can be done. But we did not apply them for the same reason that we did not test intelligence and relied on the subjective assessment of the staff. They had no doubt that some boys arrived at the hostel with a greater capacity to relate than others. We formed the opinion in the case of no fewer than eight boys that they seemed to display, on arrival, practically no capacity to establish relationships with people. One at least of these eight seemed to improve in this respect while he was at the hostel, and is now doing extremely well. Another of the eight is also doing very well, but this is because the hostel was able to put him in a position where he could make the maximum use of his talents, which were rather unusual. But the remaining six of this eight remain seriously disturbed people, about whose future it is difficult to be optimistic. On the other hand, seven boys came to the hostel with a capacity to relate which, while perhaps not quite normal, approached very nearly to it and while some of these nevertheless presented serious problems, two are now doing extremely well and others provide grounds for optimism. This leaves thirteen in the middle range, of whom about half can be seen to be making real progress.

The other symptoms we can perhaps run over more rapidly. Of not more than two or three boys could it be said that their word could be relied on, and of ten at least it must be said that their lying was well beyond anything that could be considered normal. Ten could be said to be abnormally aggressive, of whom four could be so extremely violent as to be a danger to their fellows. Nine were known to steal frequently, and in four of them, stealing assumed pathological proportions and characteristics. Seven indulged in behaviour that can only be called bizarre, for example, the boy who, with no apparent provocation, locked himself in his bedroom by pushing the heavy furniture against the door and then proceeded to throw the lighter articles out of the window; or the boy who got up in the middle of the night and paraded the streets dressed in an improvised Ku Klux Klan garb, not in any spirit of youthful prankishness, but in answer to some deeply felt need. Ten boys displayed more than usual difficulty in keeping a job.

We thus have six symptoms: difficulty in relationships, lying, aggressiveness, stealing, bizarre conduct, inability to keep a job, occurring to a serious degree 54 times among 28 boys – something like two for each boy on average. But those are only the frequently recurring symptoms. In addition there were equally serious though less frequent symptoms. These include incontinence of faeces and/or urine or the compulsive need to seek 'punishment' by persistently provoking people. Furthermore, all the symptoms listed above were liable to appear in a minor degree among boys with whom they were not a major symptom: many lied or stole beside those who did so seriously, a few were sporadic enuretics. Finally there is a large group of symptoms less serious socially than those hitherto mentioned, but none the less indicative of emotional disorder. These were such things as excessive food fads, attention seeking, insomnia and its opposite, excessively heavy morning sleeping, obsessive tidiness or the compulsive need to create disorder, and so on.

It will be recalled that one of the criteria for admission was that the applicant should have made some progress towards stability and in giving a picture of the kind of boy we received, it is necessary to see how far this condition was met. In this we had to rely largely on the opinion of the headmaster. He would normally guard against the danger of mistaking adjustment to the *mores* and regime of the school with growth towards stability, by checking his observations against what was learned about the boys' behaviour during holiday periods. The kind of boy who came to us however presented unusual difficulties in making this comparison. If he went home, allowances had to be made for the exceptionally chaotic and hostile atmosphere of most of 'our' boys' families. Many of them did not go home but to holiday placements which were liable to vary from year to year and which therefore did not supply a reliable yardstick. These circumstances made it more difficult than usual for those concerned with the boy during his school years to make a sound assessment about progress towards stability, and in the event they were often mistaken.

In expressing an opinion therefore about the degree to which this criterion proved to have been met, it should perhaps be made clear that in no case is any criticism of the schools implied. The headmaster was denied our opportunity to get a clear picture of his boy apart from the regime and circumstances to which he had become accustomed at the school.

So far as could be judged from a perusal of case histories and an observation of the boys after arrival at the hostel, there seemed to be nine boys of the twenty-eight stayers in whom no appreciable change could be seen between the time of their entry to the school and the time of their admission to the hostel; but in no fewer than six of these cases there was clearly a very good adjustment to the school. This means that of the twenty-eight boys, two-thirds were seen to have been to a greater or lesser degree helped by the school and presumably they, as well as the nine who did not seem to have been helped, would have become very much worse if they had never been to a school for maladjusted children. It must be said, however, that the amount of help derived was in some cases very little, and only four seem to have received outstanding help.

In no circumstances, of course, is this to be taken as a general judgement on the value of schools for maladjusted children. It refers only to a small group of the most difficult boys, selected because they seemed unlikely to succeed without further help.

CHAPTER FOUR

THE HOUSEMEETING

A description and discussion of the work of the housemeeting follows not because it is the most important aspect of the work of the hostel, which is, rather, to be found in the next chapter than in this one, but because it is frequently referred to. It must be said, however, that although the staff did not give it first priority in this sense, the residents probably did, and it may well be the feature of the hostel's life most obvious to the casual visitor. Certainly it seems unusual to the uninformed visitor if he has been indoctrinated with the ancient assumption that the young should always defer to their elders and that their elders should exercise unquestioned authority over them.

At Reynolds House I, who have preached freedom for the young all these years, made attendance at the housemeeting compulsory. This seems inconsistent. But in the first place, the young men who came to us, like their elders and betters, had long suffered the customary indoctrination about authority, that the lives of the young should be governed by their elders, and that they should bow to authority; because authority knows best. They had been fairly successfully indoctrinated and, like Robert Tressal's *Ragged Trousered Philanthropists* who saw no need for trade unions, they saw no need for any housemeeting. Furthermore, and paradoxically, shared responsibility deprived them of one of the major satisfactions of youth, that of kicking against the pricks. How were they to rebel against authority if they were their own authority? I am not concerned at this moment to argue whether or not it is a good thing for the young to have an authority to rebel against; I am merely saying that this was one of the reasons, not conscious of course, why the young men who came to Reynolds House in its early days tended to be on arrival unenthusiastic about the housemeeting.

The next point is that these young men differed from others in one important respect; their experience of life so far had been such as to make them somewhat cynical about the good intentions of adults, and mistrustful of their sincerity. This attitude may have been somewhat ameliorated by their experience in a good school for maladjusted children, but not as much, nor as often, as one would wish. Indeed, some of them had actually had experience of something that passed for shared responsibility, in which the young were allowed to decide anything they liked, so long as the adults liked it too, and indeed to make rules which the adults made them keep but which the adults felt no compulsion to keep themselves. This was bogus and they knew it to be bogus. They just took it for granted that ours would be equally bogus, so they were little interested in it.

I believe shared responsibility to be of enormous value in what Aichhorn called 'the therapy of the dis-social', but no medicine is any good unless the patient swallows it. And no meetings are of any value unless someone attends them. In a larger community it would not matter if there were a few absentees, and I have never before tried to compel people to come to meetings, though the meeting has sometimes done so; but the kind of meeting we had in mind simply will not work with less than a dozen or so, and as our total complement was a dozen everyone had to come.

In a school or similar institution the head can, if he so wishes, make the meetings part of the school programme, so that by attending a meeting the resident is losing none of his 'own' time, and might otherwise have been doing something much less amusing; but at our hostel we had to have the meetings in the young men's spare time, and they were competing with television. The time did come when we were able to compete successfully even with that insidious enemy of everything else, that surreptitious blotter-up of time; but that was after the boys had learned the value of the meeting, and how could they ever learn its value if they never attended it? So I told each boy before he came that a condition of residence at Reynolds House was that he should attend the meeting, which was held once a week at whatever time and day the meeting agreed upon. During the first year or so there was much groaning and grumbling about the waste of time, much moaning about 'Why do we have to come to the bloody meeting?' But one of the most clamant questions when it came to be realized that my retirement was drawing near was 'Will the new Warden let us have a meeting?' I told them that if they valued the meeting and were determined to keep it, the new Warden couldn't stop them if he tried. But however highly they valued the meeting, and they did come to value it highly, the less stable, the more irresponsible among them would always tend to give immediate satisfactions like a good TV programme priority over long-term gains and the public good. There would thus be almost always a few absentees, and a few absentees from so small a number would have been fatal.

Hence, then, this apparently inconsistent piece of compulsion. But it was a piece of compulsion that was voluntarily entered into because it was carefully explained to prospective residents before they applied for admission, and if the idea was too repellent, then they need not apply.

What then *was* this thing to which I attached so much importance? It had a latent purpose and a manifest purpose. The manifest purpose was that aspect of the meeting which was clearly visible and comprehensible to the residents; the latent purpose was one which was less obvious, and less comprehensible to them – most of them indeed were hardly aware of its existence – it was a therapeutic purpose. The manifest purpose, like the manifest content of our dreams, was that upon which the latent purpose hung, the medium through which the latent, or therapeutic purpose expressed itself. Of course we could have made the latent purpose clear to the residents, and they could have met together as the patients do in some psychiatric hospitals with the clearly understood purpose of discussing together their emotional problems. We chose not to do so. I have been using shared responsibility for about thirty-five years, since well before the term 'therapeutic community' came into use. But I have always soft-pedalled its therapeutic aim and loud-pedalled its practical, manifest purpose. The group methods used in mental hospitals I believe to be inappropriate for the kind of people I have been concerned with, but to maintain the flow of my narrative I defer my reasons for this to the end of the chapter.

The ostensible purpose of the housemeeting, as all the boys are told, is to watch over the implementation of Rule One, which is merely a paraphrase of the Golden Rule. Of course this could have been done by the staff; but our aim was to encourage adult standards of conduct, a mature attitude to life. There are already far too many people whose lives are governed by what 'They' say, whose standards of right and wrong, so far as they have any, are legalistic rather than moralistic. I want the young – and everyone else – to pursue the right and the good because they are right and good, and not because someone in authority compels them. The first step towards that happy state is to provide machinery by which all may criticize the conduct of any, and the community may by discussion determine what kinds of behaviour are acceptable. Those in authority, like myself and my colleagues, are also human, we may do things that the residents consider undesirable, and it is right and fair that our conduct too should be open to discussion and correction.

The housemeeting, which met normally on Sundays after midday dinner, was a completely egalitarian, democratic body which it is true had to fall back on the unsatisfactory technique of counting heads for some of its decisions, but in which all had an equal say, and if one man's, or woman's, opinion was more valued than another's, it was because of the respect which that person had earned as a member of the community.

The following is an account of a typical meeting. The agenda might read something like this (it had been hastily scribbled on a bit of paper by the Secretary just as the meeting was assembling):

1 Minutes of previous meeting
2 Matters arising from minutes
3 Norman – bedroom
4 Christopher – TV
5 D. Wills – Horace ('D. Wills' because we generally had several Davids)
6 Hubert – shirt
7 Elizabeth – laundry
8 Treasurer's report
9 Workshop report.

The first item calls for no comment. In the early days there were no minutes, but they began to be kept as the need for them was seen. They were atrociously kept for a year or two, after that they were very well maintained. Arising from the minutes there might have been a couple of items like this:

SAM, RADIO

At the previous meeting Jim had complained that his radio had disappeared for several days and had then been found beside Sam's bed. It transpired in discussion that Sam had 'borrowed' it and had been taking it to work every day. Sam was a depressed youth with inferiority feelings who had been using this device to court popularity among his workmates, and this point (though not in that language) would have been made in extenuation by one of the adults at the last meeting, while residents would have expressed the customary horror of offences against property. The meeting had eventually told Sam that he must give Jim 2s 6d towards the cost of new batteries, and Sam was now being asked whether he had done so. He had said last week, as residents in such a position often did, with a great deal of offensive language, that *he* wasn't going to pay any half-crown, and the meeting couldn't make him, and Jim knew what he could do with his so-and-so radio. But that was a week ago and, again following a common pattern, when he had calmed down he had duly paid. It did sometimes happen on such an occasion that the offender had so far committed himself to a refusal to pay that he could not bear the loss of face involved in climbing down, and it would transpire at the next meeting that he had not paid. More ill-temper and bad language would ensue, but there was a little trick up my sleeve which rarely failed to solve the problem. I would offer to lend the offender the sum involved. If this offer were accepted (and it usually was) I would then hand the money over to the plaintiff, so that the offender was left with the less shaming task of repaying me in private. It is interesting to observe that even in the heyday of the meeting, residents continued to take at its face value any violent declaration of refusal to do as the meeting said, and would want to start discussing how the offender was to be coerced, until an adult would say 'Why not wait until next week, and see what's happened in the meantime?' Only twice in the five years was there a persistent defiance of the meeting. In each of these cases I eventually had a word in private with the boy concerned, pointing out to him that if he persisted in defying the governing body in this way, they would clamour for his removal, which would place me in a very embarrassing position.

The next item arising from the minutes might be:

LARRY, WASHING-UP

Washing-up was the responsibility of the males of the household (that is, washing the dishes after dinner seven days a week, and high tea on Saturdays and Sundays), and was organized by the housemeeting. The requirement to do this had not been laid upon the males by me as a compulsory duty, but by the housemeeting on my initiative. In the early days of the hostel, when there were very few boys, my deputy and I had done it all between us. When numbers grew I asked the meeting whether they knew of any reason why we should do it all, and why the other males should not also take a turn. This they cheerfully agreed to do because they saw that it was not a case of a lowly chore being done by the lower orders, so the meeting took it on and drew up a rota.

Dishwashing is to me an outward and visible sign of a certain inward and spiritual grace. It is difficult to hit upon a single word to describe this grace; the nearest I can get (and it is very inadequate) is egalitarianism, the absence of any assumption of superiority. I have held for many years that effective therapeutic work cannot be carried out, in a residential setting anyway, nor a useful relationship established, whether therapeutic, social, or educational, if the 'worker' thinks of himself as being superior to the 'client'. The person who considers it beneath his dignity to stand at the sink with his clients washing dishes, is not the sort of person I have ever wanted as a colleague of mine. I am happy to say that the members of the Reynolds House Committee, by and large, shared this view, and it was no uncommon thing to find the Chairman of the Committee engaged in this chore. So we all help with the dishes. Which brings us back to:

MATTERS ARISING – LARRY, WASHING-UP

We had very little trouble over chores at Reynolds House. But occasionally somebody – anyone – would go out and forget to provide a substitute, and Larry had done that very thing. To protect ourselves, my deputy and I had a standing arrangement that we would substitute for each other, but Larry had not been so careful. The meeting had long since ordained that if a substitute had to be found at the last minute for a defaulter, the defaulter had to pay him 1s 3d. Larry was now being asked whether he had paid his 1s 3d. Larry had, so the meeting spent little time on this item.

We then come to:

ITEM 3 NORMAN, BEDROOM

Norman was a rather small, rather new boy who wanted to move from his bedroom (there were three boys to a bedroom) to another. This was usually done with very little fuss if the person who wanted to move could find someone who was willing to swap places with him and if their respective stable companions raised no objections. Norman had been unable to find anyone who was willing to change with him. It appeared that Harold, a big and rather aggressive older boy had adopted such an unpleasant domineering attitude to Norman that his life in the bedroom had become intolerable. Harold was spoken to very plainly by a number of residents and was formally rebuked by the Chairman on behalf of the meeting, and it must be said that Harold, who was not unaware of his failing, received all this with praiseworthy meekness. But Norman resolutely refused to spend another night in the same room. The point was then made that if Harold was the offender, surely it was he who should have to move, and not Norman. There was a cry of, 'Let's shift Harold', but though this was agreed in principle, the practice was problematic because no one wanted Harold. The long and acrimonious debate which followed was ended by Bernard saying (humorously, but not without a certain sanctimoniousness) that he was willing to suffer for the common good, and if Hubert was willing, as he had said, to go into Norman's room, he, Bernard, would suffer Harold in Hubert's place. In the course of this discussion a number of important lessons were learned, or at least, a step was made towards learning them; they would have to be repeated several times before they were learned by some people. Harold was beginning to learn that unless he wanted to be unpopular all his days, he would have to exercise control over his domineering manner. This was a point that could be brought home in our kind of environment. He had been for a good proportion of his life in schools for maladjusted children and other residential establishments of one kind or another without even beginning to learn it. In those establishments there was no means by which Harold's victims could defend themselves, and no way by which public opinion could be expressed. On the contrary, it is the common practice in such places for the weak to toady to the strong, and the strong often encourage each other in their sorties against the weak, so that a boy like Harold actually begins to get the impression that he is positively liked. At a place like Reynolds House where no one need fear to say exactly what he thinks, the Harolds of this world soon get the cold-shoulder. I do not assert that there is never any deferring to the bullies for the sake of a quiet life; it is less trouble even at Reynolds House to give way over some minor matter than to make a fuss and resist. But no domineering bully will ever get the impression, as they often do in more authoritarian places, that any-one ever likes him any the better for it. After all, in an authoritarian establishment the authority is maintained by the same kind of means that Harold used to get his own way in his bedroom. Where violence is used (even as a very last resort) to defend the good, the true and the right – and the establishment – it is quite possible for the young to get hopelessly confused about the whole business and to assume that because violence and authority are on the side of the right, then those who use violence and attempt to arrogate authority to themselves as Harold did in the bedroom, are therefore on the side of the right; that violence and authority *are* the right, and should be deferred to always.

For this very reason it was not by any means easy to reach the state of affairs where the bullies were cold-shouldered, and formally rebuked at the housemeeting. During the first eighteen months the house-meeting was quite ineffectual in this matter, and violence was only kept under by the unhappy expedient of my expelling two very bad offenders. The housemeeting did not really get a grip on the matter until I myself had a charge of assault successfully brought against me.

I lost my temper one night, or rather in the early hours of the morning, because I was kept awake by people racketing about the house when they should have been asleep, or at least quiet. In desperation I went to see what was going on and found a young man in his pyjamas on the half-landing. When I asked him what the devil he was up to he told me such flagrant lies and talked such arrant nonsense that I simply went right off the handle and punched his silly head. I do not know which of us was the more surprised! I was then kept awake for the rest of the night, not by external noises, as the house was from then on unnaturally silent; but by the internal discord of my own remorse.

The next day was Sunday and I said to the boy concerned that of course he would bring a complaint against me. Not at all; he had been an infernal nuisance, had got his head punched, and it had served him right. He resolutely refused to bring a complaint because, in his view, I had been perfectly justified in punching his head. So I had to bring the complaint myself. Everyone else insisted that I had been perfectly right to clobber Michael, and it was only with the greatest difficulty that I was able to convince the meeting that no one had the right to be judge and executioner in his own cause, and that if they allowed me to 'get away with it' they would be at the mercy of anyone who was big enough and brutal enough to throw his weight about; that the meeting would no longer be a democracy because people would vote as the bullies told them. Eventually they told me to give Michael 5s by way of compensation. This happened to be just the sum that Michael owed me, so we were quits.

Although I regretted having struck Michael, the eventual outcome was satisfactory. It was clear to the residents that if the meeting could make the 'boss' pay 5s. to someone for hitting him, they could do the same to anyone else and they quickly did so. If any occasion arose when it seemed possible that someone might be getting let off too lightly, I would put on a great air of injured innocence and say 'What's this then? *I* had to pay Micky five bob for clouting him under enormous provocation, and this chap . . .' From that moment bullying practically disappeared. I do not mean that no one ever struck a blow in anger, there was another occasion when I did so myself. But it was very rare for anyone to seek deliberately to get his own way by threat or violence. Nor do I mean that they were prevented by fear of having to hand over some money. I mean that it was realized that if the meeting could and would go to that length, then the meeting must be serious in its objection to violence. The punishment was seen to be what in fact punishment of this kind is; society's expression of moral condemnation of certain kinds of behaviour. It was not until people were made to pay damages for violence that the violent realized that there really was a strong public opinion against them, and it was the public opinion rather than the penalty that really brought about a change. By the time Harold had come among us with his domineering ways, public opinion was strong enough to be effective. Harold was very severely rebuked and took his rebuke meekly, as well as his change of bedrooms.

The next item was:

ITEM 4 CHRISTOPHER, TV

Christopher complained that the TV reception was lousy, and this was because we had such a crummy aerial (it was an ordinary V-shaped internal aerial). I ventured to express the inexpert view that reception might be better if a) the aerial were not mishandled, and b) people would mess about less with the controls of the set. This view was shouted down and the deputy Warden, who knew about electronics, said there was some truth in both points of view. There was a long discussion and a few weeks later the meeting spent £5 of its money on a set of loft aerials which the deputy Warden and some of the boys erected. Although NAMH provided things like radio, record players, workshop tools and so on for the amusement and entertainment of the residents, they were maintained by the housemeeting.

ITEM 5 DAVID WILLS, HORACE

Horace had been in breach of the ten-thirty rule, having been out until after eleven without leave. A little explanation is perhaps called for here, because, as the 10.30 rule was not made by the housemeeting, there was no reason why they should be held responsible for it. In fact I never insisted that they should, but had sought their help. The line I had taken had been this: acceptance of this rule, like attendance at the housemeeting, was a condition of residence at the hostel, which all had understood and accepted before they came. There was, therefore, a kind of contract between each resident and the Warden. Horace had now broken his contract, which was thus no longer binding on me, so I need no longer keep Horace at the hostel. Obviously, however, I was not going to throw poor old Horace out just because he came in late one night, so I put this point to the meeting and asked them whether they would care to devise some action that would help Horace to remember that he had after all agreed to this rule, and thus relieve us both of an embarrassing situation. This attitude was accepted and understood by the meeting, and their usual line was to say, 'Not to ask for late leave for one week', though persistent offenders might be more severely dealt with. One such persistent offender was fined as much as £2 – and paid it. It is true that I might myself have imposed some small penalty, but I did not do so for several reasons. One was that there was much value in discussing these matters publicly, which meant that everyone was from time to time reminded of his undertaking to accept this rule, and opportunities were provided for reiterating the reasons for it. More importantly, penalties imposed arbitrarily by one person in authority are rarely unaccompanied by secret or expressed grievances connected with alleged unfairness or discrimination. If the meeting dealt with the matter, not only was justice done, but justice was manifestly seen to be done.

Item 6 Hubert, Shirt

Hubert complained that one of his shirts had disappeared. This was a constantly recurring complaint. They usually turned up eventually, and sometimes the borrower was identified and made to pay compensation. On one occasion when a valuable new shirt which had been a present disappeared in this way and had not turned up after some weeks the meeting bought the boy another one, but they wisely did not make a practice of this.

Item 7 Elizabeth, Laundry

Another hardy perennial. 'Will residents *please* remove their clean laundry from the hall table because there's a lot more waiting to go on and there's no room for it.' It was placed there because nothing would persuade some boys to get their new clothes marked, when it would have been distributed to their beds. This problem became such a nuisance that eventually the meeting inaugurated a system by which any clothes still on the table after Sunday dinner were auctioned off after the meeting!

Item 8 Treasurer's Report

The meeting had long since decided that it needed funds, and everyone was required to pay a shilling a week. Although the elected treasurer sometimes had a little difficulty in extracting the shillings from the boys, I was surprised by the constancy with which this fund was maintained. Sometimes months would elapse without a penny being spent, and I could not understand why someone did not say, 'Wotthehell do we pay this bob a week for? I propose we drop it.'

But no-one ever did. We have just seen one use to which the funds were put when the meeting bought new aerials for the TV. They were also used to provide games for the quiet room, for example, they bought a dictionary for the Scrabble-players (because the *Pocket Oxford* kindly given by the Chairman of the Reynolds House Committee was not considered good enough); to maintain the tools in the workshop; to finance holiday outings and parties. If there was any wanton or unnecessary damage to property I presented the meeting with a bill which they usually paid, and would then perhaps recoup from the offender if they could identify him, which they usually could without much difficulty. The balance was generally between £5 and £15, and while the books were badly and inaccurately kept, errors usually seemed to be on the right side, i.e. more money in the kitty than there should be, not less.

ITEM 9 WORKSHOP REPORT

As the workshop was provided for the benefit of the residents, the meeting appointed a workshop steward to look after it, to try to keep it tidy and to keep an eye on the tools. He reported each week to the meeting. More often than not his report would consist of the duo-syllable 'Sallright'. Sometimes he would report that a tool was missing and if it could not be found someone would be authorized to buy a replacement. The only other matter that gave rise to feeling about the workshop was when someone dismantled his motor-cycle there, and then lost interest, leaving his property so strewn about the place that it was almost impossible to get in, much less use it.

It will be seen that the uses and virtues of the meeting were many. At a severely practical level it dealt with minor disciplinary problems, and some major ones, in a way that eliminated charges of unfairness and discrimination which can so often arise when these are dealt with by one person in authority. The judgement of one's peers is more easily acceptable and more meaningful than the dictates of an adult. In the process the fact was repeatedly brought home by experience that society has to make rules, or come to agreements, as the house-meeting did, for the convenience and protection of its members, and experience showed how all could be adversely affected by the delinquencies of one. Something was learned of tolerance, of understanding others' points of view, as well as of committee procedure, and everyone, even the weakest and smallest, was able to 'stick up for himself', and effectively too, against any would-be tyrant. All these benefits are obvious, and they arise from the 'manifest' purpose or function of the meeting. But there were other benefits, less obvious, arising from the latent function. The discussions, sometimes long and involved, about people's behaviour, provided opportunities to learn how we are all influenced in some measure by impulses and motives other than those of which we are immediately aware, and while specific interpretations of an individual's actions were rarely given, and psychiatric terminology rigorously eschewed, generalized interpretations of certain kinds of behaviour could from time to time be given, and there were many opportunities for the percipient and enlightened adult to prod a youth, by oblique remarks, by gentle insinuation or by downright challenge, to examine his own motives, and to make allowances for people acting under the stress of emotional disturbance. This was an important function of the housemeeting, and by no means all contributions of this kind came from the adults. Boys sometimes helped each other, and it was not uncommon for an adult to have *his* motives brought into question. The great point was that those motives could be questioned, frankly and openly instead of furtively and subversively in the bedrooms at night. This leads to the last virtue of the housemeeting to which reference will be made, though there are many others, it had considerable cathartic value. If a meeting were unduly noisy and heated, with vituperation in all directions, with the chairman (usually one of the boys) vainly shouting for order while perhaps some were only with difficulty restrained from physical assault on each other – after such a meeting the staff always knew that they could look forward to a quiet, relaxed, Sunday evening. But that was not the only value of this cathartic exercise. Knowledgeable visitors would quite often comment on how well the furniture and fittings had stood up to years of supposed assault by maladjusted adolescent boys. The reply was a simple one. There was no need to take it out on the furniture because ample opportunity was provided for the boys legitimately to take it out on each other, and the staff, at the weekly housemeeting. The meeting minimized frustration, and frustration is very bad for furniture.

To the residents, however, the housemeeting became, in spite of its discouraging start, an essential and integral part of their living together. They came to see it as the protector of their liberties, the means by which oversight could be given to the observance of that fundamental rule upon which the communal life was based, that we should do as we would be done by. Frequently in discussions I would remind the meeting of a favourite passage of mine from Chesterton: 'If you break the big laws you do not get liberty, you do not even get anarchy. You

get the small laws.' This passage had immediate relevance to our condition and our circumstances and the more sober and intelligent among
the residents at least, were able to see that the degree to which they
were able to maintain the observance of the one 'big law' was the degree
to which the hostel could maintain its freedom from all the little pettyfogging prohibitions and restrictions.

Finally I return to the question of why, for the kind of boys we
had at Reynolds House, I think it desirable that much of the therapeutic process should be carried on unobserved and unrecognized by
them and without their conscious participation.

I am a great believer in freedom. I accept Rousseau's ringing
assertion at the beginning of his *Social Contract* that man is born free
and is everywhere in chains. We are born free, and we constantly seek
to enslave ourselves, always seeking to put the blame on something
or somebody else, constantly pursuing a different kind of determinism,
from Calvinism to Communism. Calvin, if I understand him aright
(and he is a bold man who claims that he does), said that our fate
throughout eternity was fore-ordained by divine fiat, and we are all
slaves of the doctrine of election. Some centuries later, biologists began
to examine our inheritance, and began to cry that we were slaves to
that – we became what our genes made us. We are slaves, said others,
to our environment and upbringing and can never be anything but
what our environment makes us. Marx – who, if I remember rightly,
had the impertinence to quote Rousseau – was quite sure that we are
entirely the creatures of economic circumstances, and are what
economics make us. Then there were the psychologists who tell us
that we are helplessly driven by our instincts, and what we are and
become depends entirely on unconscious forces that we cannot control;
we are what the id and superego make us. I say nothing of the
behaviourists who are now gaining ground again and who assure us
that we are what our conditioning makes us. Well, clearly they cannot
all be right, but I venture to suggest that they *can* all be wrong, and
it is my profound conviction that they are. Our lives, I believe, *can*
be determined by any of these forces if we are willing to be enslaved,
but equally we can rise above them all. There was a verse of W. E.
Henley's which in the innocence of my adolescence I used to declaim –

> It matters not how strait the gate
>   How charged with punishment the scroll
> I am the master of my fate
>   I am the captain of my soul.

Every one of these various determinists has assured me at one time or another that those lines are sentimental nonsense, but I utter them now with equal conviction in my maturity, with half a century's further experience of life.

One of the greatest wrongs we can do to the young in our care is to allow them to get the idea that they are as they are because of things that happened to them in their earlier years. It is true that those things did happen, and may profoundly influence their lives. *Our* knowledge of this fact helps us to understand and to sympathize, it helps us to be patient and forgiving, it helps us to be non-punitive in our attitude. But let us not encourage young people to be too patient and long-suffering with *themselves*! History teems with examples of people who suffered such deprivations in their childhood and rose above them, as with our help, our kind of youngster may. I never come nearer to despair than when some maladjusted youth says to me '*I* carn elpit. Look at the way I was brought up.' There are few greater tragedies than those of maladjusted young people who are convinced that they can never be otherwise because they have been enslaved for all time by their upbringing. The reason it is so great a tragedy is that so often that idea is implanted in their minds by people like myself, seeking to be helpful and understanding. A bad start can be a challenge; let us not make it a shackle. So that is why I soft-pedal the therapeutic purpose of our housemeeting, and loud-pedal its practical, day-to-day aspects. I am not saying that I pretend the therapeutic purposes are not there; only that I do not push them to the forefront, and I do not believe it is necessary to shout about them in order to make use of them.

CHAPTER FIVE

STAFF ROLES AND ATTITUDES

Apart from providing for the physical needs of the residents, the aim of the staff was to create an environment that was conducive to growth; growth that is towards maturity and towards greater stability. Growth towards maturity is a natural process, but it can be helped or hindered by environment. In the same way, every living organism has an innate tendency towards wholeness, and the sick organism tends to be self-healing if the environment is not hostile. At Reynolds House we believed that the main essential elements of a milieu conducive to the encouragement of these natural propensities are three in number: warmth, security and freedom. By warmth is meant, of course, in this context emotional warmth, though physical warmth is no less important; the hostel was always kept very warm and very well-lit. The general atmosphere and régime was one that was designed to provide these elements, but there were constantly present also certain kinds of stimuli. It is proposed to say something about the general climate and conduct of the house before going on to speak of these more specific aids to development, which of course included the housemeeting.

This climate was in general one of easy egalitarian informality, though not that extreme permissiveness where 'anything goes'. This word 'permissiveness' causes a lot of trouble. I mean by permissiveness simply that while I consider it quite proper to hold out to people what I conceive to be desirable standards of conduct, I do *not* believe that any good purpose is served by my compelling them to adopt my standards by the fear of sanctions. I am perfectly happy about 'do not spit'; what I jib at is the 'penalty forty shillings'. The critical reader may say, 'Only a few pages ago you were telling us of a boy being fined this very sum, as if it was something of a triumph', but the inconsistency is not as great as it may seem to be. The willingness of the housemeeting to impose a penalty on one of their number, and by inference contingently upon themselves, is evidence of the acceptance of responsibility for the common good, which is a step in an educative process in which the next step, one hopes, is the willingness of the individuals constituting the housemeeting each to pursue that good for its own sake, and not out of fear of sanctions. My own personal unwillingness to threaten punishment arises from assuming that the person to whom I am talking has already reached the stage where he cares for the right for its own sake. To make that assumption is, I believe, one way of helping to create such an attitude in the person concerned. It arises also from the fact that at Reynolds House the responsibility for the maintenance of such rules as we had lay in the hands of the community as a whole, and not in mine personally. I am not among those who believe that the young should never be told what their elders believe to be right and good, but neither would I compel acceptance of those standards. This is permissiveness as used at Reynolds House.

It was, then, a régime of easy, egalitarian informality, and permissiveness in the sense described. Christian names were commonly used but not insisted upon. Few things are more ridiculous than the insistence of a middle-aged man that the young should address him by his Christian name, though I do not think that quite as absurd as the same man insisting that he should be 'Sirred' and 'Mistered'. Anyone was perfectly at liberty to call any members of the staff anything he liked. My wife was called variously, Liz, Elizabeth, Willsy, or Mrs Wills, largely, it seemed, according to the mood of the person addressing her. Her deputy, Mrs Skilton, was invariably Mrs S., or simply, S. The deputy Warden was called by a diminutive of his Christian name, though one holder of the office had a nickname. Like my wife, I enjoyed various forms of address. Some called me David, some Wills, or Willsy (rather confusing at times as some addressed my wife in that way), while others never addressed me, throughout the length of their stay, otherwise than as Mr Wills. This I am sure was according to their needs. It may well be that those who saw in me an ego-ideal for their own adoption would naturally want that ideal to be one that was respected, and therefore called me Mr Wills; others, using me as an external super-ego, would want to convince themselves that this authority figure was not after all one to be dreaded and feared, and therefore addressed me more familiarly. But this is speculative. We commonly addressed the boys by whatever name they customarily used themselves, and here again there was no rule. While our tendency at first was to use a boy's Christian name, some came in time to be called by nicknames, and some, for no reason that I have been able to fathom, by their surnames.

It will thus be seen that the common outward forms of respect often insisted on by, for example, teachers and child-care officers, were not insisted on by us. We held that whether the staff were 'respected' (in this superficial sense) or not was of little real importance. But we did feel it to be of absolutely vital importance that the residents should feel that *they* were respected, and not merely in that superficial sense, because this can be the beginning of that self-respect in which many of them were lacking. Our aim therefore, was to expect from them a return of that basic respect for their person, property, feelings, liberties and opinions which they received from us. Naturally, we felt ourselves to be bound by that first rule which I had explained to postulants for admission, and it was made clear that staff and boys alike had an equal right of complaint when they felt that rule to have been breached to their disadvantage. Thus undue noise in the bedrooms late at night was not an offence against discipline, as it is regarded in many such places, it was an infringement of other people's right to sleep, though it must be admitted that by and large this right was more precious to the older than to the younger members of the community.

An important and essential corollary of this kind of informality was the readiness to express one's feelings, and we did not feel ourselves, boys or adults, to be inhibited in the expression of those feelings. It is true that in the main the usages of polite society came more readily to the staff than to the residents, but when anger was aroused, it was usually expressed, and it was not unusual for me to 'blow my top' at a boy whose behaviour had been particularly offensive. It was even more common for boys to do the same, though their expressions of anger (or ill-temper) were perhaps more often from latent and irrational causes than from manifest and rational ones. The great point was that they felt as free as I did to express those feelings, and there was no question of repeating the situation so many of them had been confronted with at school, in which it was perfectly in order for a staff-member to abuse a boy, but impertinence for the boy to use the same kind of words to the adult.

Food is important to all of us and often has a great deal of emotional significance to maladjusted young people. Many of them had been troublesome in infancy over feeding, and very often difficulties in the parent-child relationship were first expressed in feeding problems. If the feeding battles that take place between child and mother are not resolved they are apt to be repeated in the relationship between adolescent and mother-figure. Hence, although the food at Reynolds House was beyond any doubt exceptionally good, and this was the universal view of our many visitors, there was a great deal of grousing about it, some of it highly offensive and emotionally charged. 'What's this muck then? You don't expect me to eat this shit do you?' And there were very many food-fads. These were pandered to by our long-suffering womenfolk with a degree of care and patience far exceeding what I should have been able to deploy, and I found myself from time to time growling like an impatient father at the way the residents were fussed over. But this was all perfectly natural and proper and had the desirable effect of enhancing our respective roles as mother-figure and father-figure. There were two or three boys in particular who never sat down to an evening meal without giving us a critique of the dishes placed before them, and it became a standing joke among the other residents who, as soon as one of these boys sat down, would wait expectantly for their unfavourable comments. As a rule we were able to ignore their remarks or laugh at them, though there were occasions when my patience, and even, very, very rarely, that of my wife, was exhausted and I would 'blow my top'. But those occasions were rare.

Of course, everyone had their meals together, though in practice the evening meal and midday dinner at weekends were the only ones at which the whole community was likely to be assembled. Breakfast was a movable feast eaten in the kitchen. The boys were called at different times, according to the time they had to be at work, and were given breakfast when they came down. Most of the boys had their lunch out, but the evening meal was served with a certain measure of formality, and civilized behaviour was expected. The large refectory tables were arranged to make three sides of a square. One of my colleagues sat at each of the 'free' ends and my wife and I sat at the middle of the connecting table. This was done so that the family could eat *as* a family and conversation would be general. For our purposes small formica-topped tables that would have made the place look like a café, were 'out'. Whereas bad language in moderation was tolerated in the house so long as there were no women within earshot, and was not bawled at the top of one's voice, it was objected to when women were present, and always at mealtimes. There was no rule about getting 'cleaned up' for meals, but something might be said, perhaps jocularly, and not necessarily by the staff, if someone came to the table in a filthy condition, or seemed to be making a practice of coming to the table unwashed. This was our attitude in general to personal habits and behaviour: no condemnation, no ordering about, no regulations, but a reminder of what was customary in civilized society, expressed with a degree of mildness or strength as the particular circumstances warranted. Thus when I say *this* was objected to, or *that* was discouraged, or the other was 'expected', I mean exactly what I say, and am not using polite euphemisms for orders and regulations. In our kind of régime anyone, old or young, had a right to object to anything that gave him offence, to try to discourage behaviour that he found unacceptable, and to expect people to return his courtesy. I do not deny that in the main more regard was given to my objections and my expectations than was given to some, to the objections, for example, of some loud-mouthed bully who commonly himself behaved offensively. But I believe this was because the residents had found good cause to respect me as a person, rather than because they had learned to fear me as a person in authority, and of course this was also true of my colleagues.

When the boys came home from work they were received by staff, with a cup of tea in the quiet room, though not all would want it or be in time for it. Although the purpose of this ritual was to try to reproduce the circumstances of home when the returning child seeks, though not consciously, to assure himself of the security of the parental presence, the boys in fact went about the same matter in a different way: they would burst into the house through the kitchen entrance and ask what was for dinner, before going on to the quiet room for tea or the common room for TV. The quiet room was the smaller and cosier of the two main public rooms. Guitars, non-amplified, mouth organs and so on, were often played in the quiet room because it is possible to carry on a conversation in the same room as an ordinary guitar, but not in the same room as a radio or record-player used by the modern young.

The boys (though not the staff) had their beds made for them except on the days they were not working. This is the practice in most working-class homes, and it was felt that in any case a boy who has to be at work by 7.30 a.m. or 8.00 a.m., is not likely to make much of a job of it. The impression made upon some at least of our many visitors was that the boys were over-indulged; and certainly in the matter of small personal services, such as getting a chair or an extra cup from the kitchen, the position tended to be precisely the opposite of that in many residential establishments for the young, in the sense that the staff at Reynolds House usually did for the boys the kind of things which in many establishments the boys do for the staff. Rightly or wrongly the working-class adolescent boy does very little in the home and it was thought right, by and large, for the hostel boys to enjoy the same privileges as the friends they made outside. But that is not all. I am in favour of the young performing small services for their elders if they do so spontaneously out of a desire to please. I do not want the young doing things for me because someone says they have to. I particularly do not want it in a residential establishment, because there it smacks too much of the bad old days of the Poor Law, when the Master and Matron regarded the inmates as inferior beings, and their personal servants. I am not speaking from hearsay or reading: this is something I remember. To the child brought up in a civilized environment, the small services he is asked, perhaps compelled, to do, like getting a chair for mother, are merely such as he sees his elders doing for each other from time to time, out of common courtesy. To the institution child lacking that background, they are apt to be seen more as the tribute which grown-ups exact from children, the staff from the inmates. For this reason too, then, I am anxious that our Reynolds House boys should see these small services being carried out by me and my colleagues. The effect of this was that we sometimes seemed, to the visitor, to be waiting on them hand and foot, picking up their coffee cups from the quiet room floor, fetching them ashtrays and so on. I cannot say that I saw much evidence of our example in these matters being emulated, but I cherish the hope that when in later years, in another environment, they begin to feel the need to behave like civilized people, they will recall the way the adults at Reynolds House conducted themselves, and will think of a gentleman as one who serves, rather than as one who is served.

As in any other home (though not in many other Homes), there was no 'getting-up time' on non-working days, and if a boy chose to 'lie in' he was perfectly at liberty to do so, and in so doing he exercised a liberty which we of the staff also enjoyed on *our* days off. The demand to help with the washing up, made for utilitarian and financial reasons as well as for educative ones, is not often made with success in working-class families.

One by-product of what may seem to some to be a very indulgent attitude was that there was rarely any difficulty in an emergency in getting volunteers at holiday times or other periods of domestic shortage to help with the housework, and my wife and I have come down more than once on a Sunday morning to find the whole of the ground floor cleaned up by a boy returning from a night-shift.

In some hostels, boys who are out of work are required to pay their way by doing work about the house. This we never did, though of course we never rejected offers of help from such boys. The reason for this, apart from any reasons that have already been given by implication, was simply that our boys were expected to pay for their board whether they were working or not. This is dealt with more fully in the chapter on work and wages.

A resident's time was his own when he was not at work. He was free to come and go as he pleased, without seeking anyone's permission and without telling anyone where he was going, subject of course to the rule about being in by 10.30 p.m. In consequence of this freedom, of the relaxed atmosphere, the easy relationships and the absence of anything authoritarian or inquisitorial, it was very rare indeed for the staff not to know where everyone was, and very often they would know of a boy's intention to take some unwise course early enough to dissuade him. If there had been any question of *forbidding* him, then the probability is that usually we should never have heard of the boy's intention, and there would thus have been no opportunity to forbid. Residents were free to bring their friends of either sex, but, as in any other family, the housemother liked due warning if they were coming to a meal though, again as in any other family, she did not always get it. High tea on Sundays was often a very happy occasion, when everyone had to sit with elbows well tucked in to make room for visiting boys and girls. Television, record player, radio, table tennis, the tools in the workshop, were all freely available at all times, subject only to such arrangements as the housemeeting might make for their regulation. Apart from table tennis, games were not provided because it was thought that these inexpensive items might very well be bought by the residents themselves and hence perhaps given better care. This in fact was what happened.

At 10.30 p.m. (later on Saturdays) the public rooms were vacated, doors and windows locked, ground floor lights put out and all, including the staff, retired to their bedrooms. There was never any question of dormitory supervision or lights out. Good order in the bedrooms was left to Rule One and such supplementary rules as the housemeeting might from time to time make. They made one, for example, that while bedside lights might be kept on as long as the owner wished, top lights and radios were to be switched off half an hour after bedtime.

There was no religious observance, though a fair amount of informal discussion about religion, in which I never hesitated to make my own views known; no insistence on church-going, though I did not hesitate to remind any who had, so to speak, already contracted obligations of this kind to a particular church, not that my reminders ever had the slightest effect; and there was no regulation of the residents' finances.

Such was the nature of the background against which the housemeeting operated. This too was the background against which the staff sought to establish personal relationships with the residents. These relationships, like the housemeeting, had two aspects; the provision of security, and the provision of stimulus. It is now time to discuss the nature of those relationships, and how they operated.

In discussing selection procedure, the point was made that in interviewing a prospective resident I was always very careful to avoid any reference to the possible role of the staff as parent-figures. It was assumed that the boy was eager to escape adult tutelage, was hardly aware of any need for adult support, would reject it if offered—and demand it if it were not. In the event, the last assumption was amply justified.

This demand for a filial relationship of course arose not from any conscious purpose on the part of the resident but from his unconscious needs. It began only as, and so far as, he came to accept the adults as persons of integrity and authority,[1] who were totally disinterested (but the reverse of *un*interested) and whose motives were entirely without undertones of personal advantage; persons whom nevertheless, while they were friendly and approachable, were apparently not concerned to thrust their opinions and views on him, or to order his life. When the adults were so recognized they were trusted; when they were so trusted they were used (and abused) and finally taken for granted in much the same way as, in a good family, the parents are taken for granted.

The way in which residents demanded that staff adopt a parental role is perhaps best conveyed by recounting one of the most outstanding examples. This particular incident concerned myself in my role as father figure. Although I am quite as willing as the next man to appear friendly and approachable, I have to confess that I do not very much look like that. Nature, or experience, or my own inner conflicts or something, have caused me to have a somewhat forbidding exterior, and I do not care to make a fool of myself by trying to assume a manner of false *bonhomie*. The tendency therefore was for the residents, especially when they first arrived, to see me solely as an authority figure, and to make that kind of demand upon me. The boy concerned on this occasion was Jim, who one day went to Brighton with a group of Rockers, and returned in the early hours badly scared. His friends had turned out to have more serious delinquent tendencies than he had realized. Several of them had behaved very badly, two had been arrested, and Jim was much relieved to find himself still at large.

---

[1] Authority is here used not in the sense of being *in* authority, but as being persons who clearly know 'what's what', who have no doubts about the difference between right and wrong, who quite palpably know what they are doing and where they are going.

However, a month or so later he said to me, in his most aggressive 'dare you to do your worst' manner, 'Going to Brighton tomorrow'. Such a remark, but for its belligerency, would normally have called for no more than a casual 'Ah yes? Have a nice time!' but on this occasion I felt, intuitively, that a little more was called for. So I said, 'Oh yes? Who are you going with?' He said he was going with Jerry and Fred, and Fred was taking him on the back of his bike. 'Jerry and Fred?' I said, in a ruminative kind of way, 'Those aren't the clots you went with a few weeks ago when you nearly got nicked, are they?' But they were. And Jim told me in a very aggressive way that they were good chaps, absolutely great, and what had I got against them? I said simply, 'Well, you'll be a bloody fool if you go with that lot again', and walked away.

It was clear that Jim wanted the excitement of a motor-bike ride to Brighton in the company of Rockers, but at the same time knew it would be an unwise thing to do. He wanted to be stopped from going, but the father-figure could not stop him if he knew nothing about it, so Jim took pains to see that he *did* know about it, so that he could put his foot firmly down and say 'No'. Actually, as will be seen, I did not say no. To do that, to forbid anything, to give orders, was quite contrary to the ethos of the establishment. But the opinion of authority, unequivocally expressed in the vigorous vernacular, was quite enough for Jim. He did not go.

I should like to say a little more about this before I go on to talk about the poor mother-figures, who had a much worse time of it than I ever did. To the casual observer, one with no knowledge of our habits and methods at Ryenolds House, watching this little scene and its sequel, it might seem that I had wonderful control over the residents. I just say 'I wouldn't if I were you', and they don't. What, asks that casual observer, is the form of the disciplinary system on which this control is based, what are the sanctions, what would have happened if Jim had ignored my advice?

The fact is of course that Jim took my advice because I had *no* control, in the disciplinarian sense. He could have gone, I would not have tried to stop him, there would have been no consequences when he returned: but he did not go. If, on the other hand, it had been my usual practice to impose myself as an authority figure, Jim, an adolescent, would have wanted to flout my authority. Because the authority was not imposed, it was sought and, indeed, assumed to be present in greater degree than was really the case. I had indeed only as much authority as Jim chose to invest me with, and the more he needed to be stopped, the greater the authority he gave me. He saw himself as having been forbidden, when in fact he had only been advised.

To invest me with authority in this way was quite a common thing, and I was often outrageously accused of having 'stopped' people from doing things when all I had done was, as in Jim's case, to express the opinion they sought. But the important thing is that I was endowed with this power because I waited for it. If I had attempted to assume it by ordering them about in matters concerning which they felt no need for help, or before they felt that need, then an entirely different chain-reaction would have been set in motion, and I should have met opposition and resistance, that opposition, that resistance, of the teenager, about which we hear so much.

So much, then, for the pursuit of paternal authority. The demanding of a mother-role was even more common, more obvious, and more trying to those upon whom it was made. Never was any resident wooed or inveigled into giving confidences; that again would have been quite contrary to the ethos and the method. But my wife and her deputy, while ironing or preparing a meal in the kitchen, were the repository of many confidences, about trouble at work, about parents, about girlfriends, about anything and everything. That part was relatively easy; we all love the role of confidant. But demands were also made of the kind to which mothers are well accustomed, and to which they usually accede. A boy is going to meet his girlfriend, and the shirt he 'must' wear is torn or dirty. Will Liz or Mrs S. mend or wash it *immediately*, he *must* wear it tonight. Or will they taper these jeans that he *must* wear when he goes to meet his cronies, who would scorn him (at that period) if they were not skintight. Requests, often couched almost as orders, of this kind were common, and if it was humanly possible they were granted. There again, I found myself adopting the paternal role of growling about the way the children were indulged by the womenfolk. If it were not possible, perhaps because the person concerned was in the middle of preparing a meal, then the boy might be helped to do it himself. These constant demands often at the most inconvenient moment and always with the maximum urgency, were bad enough, but the women had even worse to suffer. Many of the residents had highly unsatisfactory mothers against whom, consciously or unconsciously, they felt the most intense resentment and animosity. Very often those feelings were transferred to the present mother-figure, who was subjected to entirely irrational abuse and malediction. Joe, for example, who was devoted to Mrs S. and proud to be called her 'little man' even when he had become a massive six-footer, one day, without the faintest provocation, hurled at her a torrent of abuse in the foulest language. Then he pointed an airgun at her. It was not a child's toy, but a heavy, powerful weapon. He pointed it at her heart from a few feet away and said he would like to murder her. She was undoubtedly the recipient of this boy's death-wish against his mother, but this, while it explained the outburst, did nothing to make it any more pleasurable for her. But she knew that Joe would not have hated his mother if he did not also love her. The hating is part of the loving, and it is an essential element of the treatment in such a case to accept them both as part of the young person's needs, but to return only the love.

It is clear, then, that distressing as these experiences were, often to the point of prostration, they were evidence of real affective relationships. Relationships in which, during the 'positive' periods – *not* while guns were being pointed at the adult—if advice were given it was likely to be taken, in which the views and opinions of the adult were likely to be given great weight, in which there was every likelihood of that kind of identification with a loved person which leads to the adoption, in some measure, of his mores and his attitude to life. In such a relationship, furthermore, the percipient adult could by the dropped word, the casual hint, the oblique allusion, stimulate the young person to fresh views, new thoughts, a reconsideration of existing assumptions. Such words, such allusions, such hints, were constantly being given, by both the men and women in private conversation or public debate, among the teacups in the quiet room, over the kitchen sink, at the dining table, leading sometimes to animated, if not indeed heated, discussion. Leading also, it was hoped, in many cases to some amending of attitudes, and at least the beginning of yearnings after the good rather than the shoddy, the true rather than the expedient.

CHAPTER SIX

WORK AND WAGES

Sammy and Hubert are the two residents I remember as being nearest to actual unemployability. Hubert had seven jobs in his first nine weeks, two of which lasted only 90 minutes. I wrote to his child-care officer, pointing out that the hostel was intended for boys who, with support, could be expected to hold down a job, and that if Hubert continued like this we should have to consider whether Reynolds House was the right place for him. But it transpired that he was only finding his feet, which some boys found much more difficult than others.

Those of us who lived through the Great Depression of the thirties, find it difficult or impossible to adjust to the attitude of present-day youth to employment. We have got it firmly implanted within us that anyone who gives us a job is doing us a favour and we should be grateful to him. Not so Hubert and his friends, their line is that they are doing the employer a great favour by working for him. In those days the employer held the whip hand, now the worker is almost in that position. An employer came to see me one day because Eustace had robbed the till at the petrol filling station where he worked. I knew very well that Eustace was liable to do this kind of thing and if the employer had consulted me at the outset I should have advised him to keep on looking. But he was consulting me too late, and the damage had been done. I said 'You knew he would be handling money. Did you take up references, 'phone previous employers?' 'Good God, no,' he said, 'if we did that sort of thing we should never get anybody.'

Certainly it is a great boon to the Huberts of this world that they are not compelled to take *any* job, and be thankful, as we were. They can try their hands at half a dozen jobs, and keep on trying till they find the one that fits, as Hubert eventually did.

Sammy was quite a different kettle of fish. He knew what kind of job suited him and he had that kind of job, but was continually being sacked because he simply could not get up in the morning. Even the tolerant employer who would come round and roust Sammy out of bed himself, in the end had to confess himself beaten. And so did I. Sam eventually took to his bed almost permanently, just getting up each day in time to meet his girlfriend in the evening. He would not look for a job; when interviews were arranged for him he failed to turn up for them, he would not even claim unemployment insurance or social security benefit, and his rent got even more in arrears.

It was obvious of course from this and other signs that Sammy was sick, suffering from some acute emotional disorder, but nothing we could do or say would persuade him even to talk to our psychiatrist, much less to accept any of the various devices we suggested for dealing with his distress. When all else failed his parents offered to have him home, but he rejected that too. At last, when this had gone on for six or seven weeks, I told him that as (a) he owed so much rent and (b) he showed no interest whatever in finding the means to pay it and (c) refused to take any steps towards overcoming his condition, I had no alternative but to give him notice. I gave him a week's notice, and he continued exactly as before. When the final Saturday came, Sammy still seemed to be taking no action and towards evening I told him that unless he was out by 10.30 p.m., I should send for the police to eject him. At 10.30 I sent for the police. By Monday morning, entirely by his own efforts (though I did give him a few addresses and the money with which to pay a week's rent in advance), he had fixed himself up with lodgings and a job. He had a rather chequered career after this, but he kept in touch and up to now has just succeeded in keeping his head above water.

I may seem to have been taking a very hard line with Sammy, and I certainly felt this at the time, but there were two reasons, even apart from those I gave Sammy, why I felt there was no alternative. The first and lesser was that I did not want the residents to think of themselves as sick men, and there were several other boys who might easily have convinced themselves that they also were too emotionally disturbed to work. Another aspect of the same point is that to them, Sammy (at that time) was 'nuts', and if we kept him on, although he did no work and paid no rent, then clearly ours was a hostel for 'nut cases', from which it followed that they too were 'nut cases', the very impression we were anxious to avoid giving. The other reason was that the presence in the house of a non-worker had a very disturbing effect on the other boys. If a boy was out of work, the others would continually be asking 'Has so-and-so got a job yet?' and not in any spirit of tender solicitude. They seemed to experience great resentment when the answer was 'No'. I think one reason for this was their fear of their own anti-work tendencies. Few of them, in spite of all our efforts, had jobs that really gave them great satisfaction. And going to work every day, for these somewhat unstable people, was often a very real effort. Another reason for this resentment of the non-worker was something in the nature of sibling jealousy. The unemployed boy was in the house when the others went to work in the morning and still around the house when they returned in the evening. What had he been enjoying all day that they had been denied? They did not of course formulate this feeling in words, but they undoubtedly felt that the non-worker had been enjoying a greater share than they of the company and attention of the parent-figures, and this was something they could not accept with equanimity. They were of course not conscious of this as jealousy, anymore than they recognized as jealousy their cruelty to and open dislike of my wife's cat, and it usually found verbal expression only in a rationalized form as indignation about other people's laziness. But sibling jealousy it undoubtedly was, and for these reasons there was always apt to be more absenteeism among the others when a boy was unemployed, and if he did not soon get work it was highly probable that someone else would lose his job.

Sammy and Hubert, however, together with Michael, who had fourteen jobs in twenty months, were quite exceptional cases and although we had our problems, the work record in general was not unsatisfactory.

It will be manifest, quite apart from all that I have said above, that work played an important part in the lives of the residents and placement in suitable employment could help enormously in growth towards stability. An outstanding example of this is Tommy, who seemed so extremely depressed and disturbed that doubts began to be felt as to whether he could be kept at the hostel. After a few trial runs he was found the kind of job he wanted, first with a very sympathetic employer, and from that point went from strength to strength and is now thought of as one of the hostel's most outstanding successes. He has a responsible well-paid job with employers who think a great deal of him and has all the appearance of a mature and stable young man.

It was fortunate that the hostel was situated in an area that provided a rich variety of occupational opportunities. Although Bromley is often thought of as largely a commuter's dormitory, there is in fact a large number of small, and a small number of large factories within reach of the hostel, a large number of shops and the usual service trades like plumbing, decorating, electrical repairs and so on. Throughout the five years, only two boys travelled to London for their work.

Of course we experienced all the usual competition between low-paid apprenticeships on the one hand, and jobs with no skill but more pay on the other, and this in spite of the admirable intentions that many of them expressed on arrival. Quite a fair proportion arrived (thanks presumably to the good work of their teachers during the final year) with the determination to become apprentices and learn a trade, but changed their minds when they were faced with the financial realities, or they took an apprenticeship and later gave it up. The two outstanding, and most infuriating, examples of this were Henry and Christopher. I went to enormous trouble to get each of these boys exactly what he wanted, even after the youth employment officer had declared it to be very difficult if not impossible. One of them was duly apprenticed to a very good cabinet maker who would, without doubt, have taught him very thoroughly, and good cabinet makers are scarce. But he started him on £3 10s 0d a week, and this boy was very fond of money. After three months he found himself a shop job paying twice as much.

The other one of these two was a different kind of problem. He wanted to be a joiner, and after very much trouble I got him an apprenticeship with a builder who did pay a reasonable wage. Our young man fully accepted the fact that this would involve going to night school, but he had been a school-phobic and when the time came to register he was quite unable to face it. I used many expedients to get the horse as far as the water but nothing would make him drink at the academic stream. He was a good lad, however, and his employer was still willing to keep him on, either as a joiner's apprentice or in some other capacity but the boy, rather than admit that he was scared of school, insisted on leaving on the grounds that he did not like working out of doors – and then got a job as a van boy!

There was, however, another, quite different reason for early job changes, and one that led us to change our policy about employment. During the first year or so, Henry and Christopher were by no means the only boys for whom we made great efforts to get exactly the kind of job they said they wanted, only to find after a few weeks that they did not want this kind of job after all, without, as a rule, knowing what they did want. One reason is that boys do not realize that tinkering about at something at school, largely for amusement, is quite a different proposition from doing it for a living. Our cabinet-making boy, for example, who brought with him several articles which he had quite competently made in the school workshop, found that as a cabinet maker's apprentice he had to spend long hours sandpapering chair-legs. In the same way the boy who has enjoyed helping the cook and perhaps has made with her help an omelette or a fancy cake, is astonished and mortified to find that being apprenticed to the trade means handing utensils quickly on demand to a temperamental chef and washing them after use. About a quarter of the boys who came to us wanted to be chefs; only one achieved this ambition.

Again, we found sometimes that boys had been gently and kindly pressured into believing that they wanted a particular trade. Philip, a tall handsome, intelligent boy, was quite sure he wanted to be an auto-mechanic, so I got our good friends and neighbours to give him an apprenticeship. They suffered him for some months and after having discussed him with me on several occasions eventually said very regretfully that he clearly had no interest in his work and they could not keep him. Philip then said at length that what he really wanted to do was ladies' hairdressing, and it transpired that people at his school had convinced him that he really preferred working with engines. We got him into ladies' hairdressing, at which he was ultimately a roaring success. Then of course there were some whose ambitions were just not realistic in the sense that their symptoms militated against success in their chosen trade, or whose fantastic ambitions were a kind of compensation for their general inadequacy: Micky, for example, who could hardly add two and two together was determined to be a shop-assistant. I believe however that the principal reason that boys were disappointed with their chosen trade was none of these things but something quite different. As school-children they had been accustomed to a relatively easy daily routine, with only five hours' work a day, much of it organized in such a way as to make it as enjoyable as possible, often in pleasant or indeed beautiful surround-ings. They now had to work from eight in the morning until five or later in the evening, in a place that was ·perhaps dirty and noisy, sometimes with a brusque foreman who expected prompt obedience and no argument, and it was not easy to adjust to the new conditions. They would not realize at first that this is what working life is like, and would assume that the reason they found things so difficult was that they had chosen the wrong trade. It was quite useless to try to get them to understand this. They were totally disillusioned with joinery or electro-mechanics or whatever it was, and determined to do some-thing quite different, though they rarely knew what.

After much experience of going to great lengths to get a boy exactly what he wanted only to find that our efforts had been wasted, we adopted an entirely different policy. We refused utterly to take their expressed preference at its face value, and encouraged them instead to take for a few months some quite different job, often a blind-alley job, while they, and we, looked around. If after two or three months they still knew exactly what they wanted to do, and it was realistic, *then* we would make every effort to see that they got it. This approach met with a fair amount of success, though it had not been long in operation before selective employment tax put an end to many of the jobs we had been using for the 'breaking-in' period.

Jobs were normally obtained through the services of the youth employment officer, but however sympathetic he may have been, and he was very sympathetic, he did have a duty to employers as well as to us, and he had a reputation to maintain. So the chronic job-losers had to be helped (or driven) by the staff, as did also the boys whose exotic demands in the way of employment were beyond the scope of the youth employment officer, or would have taken up a disproportionate amount of his time. In all of this we were very much helped by employers. The attitude of many employers was a most heartening revelation. It was not normally our practice to say anything to employers about the background of a boy for whom we were soliciting employment, especially about his history of maladjustment, but by the time a boy had acquired a really bad work record, a little was sometimes said, with the result that the boy was often given a job for altruistic reasons, or in the hope that this employer would be able to demonstrate that *he* could manage him. In the same way, an employer would sometimes telephone to say he would have to get rid of a boy. I would usually agree most warmly that he had indeed no alternative in the circumstances and the boy had been lucky to have his job so long. I might then say a few words in passing about some of the boy's early difficulties, and much more often than not, without any request having been made by me, the employer would say something like, 'Poor devil, of course I knew nothing about all that. Perhaps I'd better keep him a bit longer and see if we can't make something of him.' This happened so often that I came to regard it as the normal reaction, and was even faintly surprised to get any other. But this generous, friendly, helpful approach came repeatedly from people of all kinds, and it is a great pleasure to record it.

On the whole, then, the work record was very encouraging. Of the twenty 'positive leavers', and the eight still in residence, no fewer than twenty-two have stuck to one kind of occupation and seem likely to continue in it. The remaining eight drifted from job to job not so much because they did not know what they wanted to do as because their ambitions were quite unrealistic in relation to their intelligence, their gifts, or the degree of their stability. Even they, however, in the main, paid their way so long as they enjoyed the support of the hostel, but it is not surprising to find that three of them are now in residential

F

establishments of one kind or another, one in a psychiatric hospital, one in an approved school and one in borstal.

Twenty-two boys out of twenty-eight more or less found their vocation, though one of these, a full time art student, is an exceptional case. Five worked as shop assistants, three of them sticking to a specific kind of commodity, while the other two moved around various kinds of shops. One boy was a local government clerk and two were solicitors' clerks, though one of these eventually returned to full time schooling and is now seeking a university place. One was a butcher, two were ladies' hairdressers, two were railway workers (one a driver, one a junior porter, who eventually joined the Royal Navy). There was one chef, one auto-mechanic and one van-driver's mate who afterwards became handyman at a boarding school. The remaining five were factory hands of various kinds. When one considers the high degree of emotional disturbance to which many of these boys were still subject this cannot be considered a bad record.

An examination of what the boys did with their money may be of interest. The adolescent is neither man nor boy, but sometimes one and sometimes the other, and his treatment must vary in like manner. A very common fallacy about the state of adolescence is to view it as a process of gradual change from child to adult in which the child is slowly shedding the characteristics of the one while assuming those of the other. This is entirely to misconceive the process, which is not so much one of gradual change as of a constant to-ing and fro-ing between the two states, not only from day to day but from aspect to aspect. Today he may be mature over his work and infantile in his attitude to money, tomorrow reversing these attitudes. These inconsistencies arose not only from the dual nature of the residents; the hostel too had a dual nature and a dual role. It was in some respects like a family home, and in others simply a boarding house in which an experiment in communal living was being carried out. This duality necessarily led to a duality in treatment which was bound to involve certain inconsistencies. These inconsistencies were nowhere more clearly to be seen than in the financial affairs of the residents.

It will be recalled that in talking to Tommy and his successors about what life would be like for them if they decided to go and live at Reynolds House, I encouraged them to think of themselves as free, independent, self-supporting citizens. In fact, of course, they were nothing like self-supporting. But not much can be done to replace adolescent fantasy with reality merely by word of mouth: it is better done by experience. Nor is there much profit in encouraging these young men to think of themselves as pensioners of society. I can conceive of circumstances in which it might be proper to say to a young man 'Don't forget that the rest of us are keeping you', but not these young men, not yet. Not until we have done everything in our power to give them a good start in life can we begin to take umbrage if they are unwilling to support themselves. What our residents actually paid did not even cover the cost of their bed and board, much less the services of the staff, whether therapeutic or domestic. But they paid a substantial portion of their weekly earnings, and a good deal more than most boys pay who are living at home with their parents. Our aim was to make the monetary aspects of the hostel a useful rehearsal of the circumstances in which they would find themselves in a couple of years' time when they moved on.

To proceed, then, with the inconsistencies. We made a fixed weekly charge of £3 5s 0d for board and lodging. At the end of the fourth year of the hostel's life we raised this by a pound, but what follows refers to the first four years before the charge was raised. The residents were encouraged (except when their lordly airs incensed the adults beyond endurance) to regard this weekly charge as proper payment for what they received, though not without an occasional reminder that they would never get such good value for their money anywhere else in Bromley, and not without an occasional reminder that this did not include the services of the staff, which, like the services of parents, were provided free. But now arose the first inconsistency. If payment of this £3 5s 0d left the boy with less than 30s in his pocket, then the rent (as the boys called it) was reduced to the point where that sum *was* left. If, for example, a boy earned only £4 a week, then he would only pay £2 10s 0d rent. In this sense board and lodging was treated somewhat as parents might treat it, as being dependent upon means. Here arises the next inconsistency; while it was reduced for the low earner, it was payable in full by the non-earner. That is to say, it was an absolute obligation whether a boy was working or not, as it would be if he were in ordinary lodgings. If a boy was out of work, the accumulated debt would be payable in weekly instalments according to his means after he started working again. This happened only very rarely because unemployed boys were encouraged to make use of social security benefits. This we regarded as an important part of their training, especially for those inadequate boys who were likely to be often unemployed. In such cases of course the boy would tell the officials that he had to pay £3 5s 0d a week in rent, and his supplementary allowance would be calculated on that basis. There was, therefore, no reason why an unemployed boy should not pay the full £3 5s 0d a week. We did not however demand this from a newly arrived boy who had not yet got his first job.

The average weekly bring home pay during a sample three months when the hostel was full was £6 5s 7d, and the average weekly amount paid as board and lodging was £2 19s 2d. It will thus be seen that in practice very few boys can have paid less than the standard charge of £3 5s 0d. There was only one boy during the first four years who regularly qualified for the reduced payment, and one or two others who might qualify for a few weeks at a time.

Two further inconsistencies may be referred to at this point. The above charges refer to boys who had not yet reached the age of eighteen. On reaching that age the charge went up by £1, subject to a pocket money 'bar' of £2 instead of 30s. Secondly, an effort was made to encourage apprentices by increasing to £2 the amount an apprentice might retain in his pocket. This was not a bribe to encourage boys to take up apprenticeships, as such it would have been woefully inadequate, but a recognition of the fact that an apprentice might well at seventeen be earning as little as a fifteen-year-old, and it was thought proper that he should not feel himself to be at too great a financial disadvantage in relation to his contemporaries.

All this may sound complicated, but it did not appear so to the residents, because they did not need to comprehend all the various possibilities and exceptions that might arise, but only their own circumstances; and to the great majority it was simply a matter of paying the fixed charge of £3 5s 0d. When a boy had done that the rest of his money was his own to deal with as he would.

Many hostels for teenagers have a sliding scale based on earnings, but I much prefer a definite fixed charge which, save for the rare exceptional reductions, can easily be equated to ordinary rent as paid by the boy in lodgings. There are many reasons for this. In the first place it is easily comprehensible to the boy, even the less intelligent boy, and he need never wonder whether the Warden is taking the right amount from him. Secondly it is realistic. From each according to his means is an admirable ideal, but it is not one that has yet been accepted by the society into which our young men were shortly to move. Thirdly and most important, it minimizes a feeling which is encouraged by the sliding scale that he is still a dependant, that he is not paying his way, but that 'they' are taking from him money which, as 'they' have, in his mind, all the money in the world, 'they' do not really need. In such circumstances it is handed over reluctantly, with resentment, and any possible opportunity is taken to defraud the hostel. I think it is true to say that the residents of Reynolds House paid their rent with pride and satisfaction, and the number of attempts to dodge paying what was due could be counted on the fingers of one hand.

Hostels which adopt the practice of the sliding scale commonly also use another practice which was rigorously eschewed at Reynolds House. Under this practice the boy is required to bring home his pay packet unopened and hand it to the Warden, who then opens it and does the boy's budgeting for him:

'This I take for your board and lodging; this I shall put on one side towards clothes; this will be towards holidays; this is for your fares to work next week; this is for your lunches. Here you are then, this is your pocket money.'

The policy at Reynolds House was precisely the opposite. The line, much appreciated by the boys, was simply:

'You have worked and earned this money, so it is yours to do as you like with. How much you earn and what you do with it is no business of ours except that we are concerned to see that you have enough. You have of course contracted a debt to the hostel for this week's board and lodging, which is obviously a first charge on your wages; what you do with the rest is entirely your own affair.'

They would say to me on Friday evenings, 'Want your money I suppose?' and thrust a bundle of grubby notes into my hand, often with some jest about robbing the poor, or being a Shylock, but always with ill-concealed pride in their independence. In the last few months at school the boy had been eagerly looking forward to having his own pay-packet, his own resources. It seems to me monstrous to take that from him and hand him back only cigarette and cinema money. Monstrous on humane, compassionate grounds, but monstrous also on educational grounds. There is no way of learning how to handle money except the experience of handling it. Of course a number of boys (though by no means all) grossly mishandled their money at first in spite of all the careful warnings and advice given by adults in the past, and now at the hostel, and in spite of all their own pious intentions, but that is all part of the process of learning. We made it quite clear that we were willing to help any boy with advice and with banking facilities, and there were few boys who did not at one time or another make use of this willingness. Banking facilities, as is well known, includes loans, though this aspect of banking was not pressed upon the boys. But they came to us all for a loan from time to time. Sometimes it would be a boy who had simply messed things up. He had come to the hostel well equipped with clothes, we insisted on that, because a lad with 30 or 40 shillings a week in his pocket could, with care, maintain a wardrobe, but he could not be expected to build one up. But sometimes a boy had simply 'blued' his money week after week for months. Then one day he realized that he must have new jeans or a pair of shoes, and in desperation came to one of us for a loan. We did not make it easy. Sometimes negotiations were abruptly ended with an 'All right, bugger yer. Yer know where you can stuff yer bloody money', though negotiations would often be taken up again, somewhat shamefacedly, a few days later. If we did lend in these circumstances it was made very clear that we were making the loan because we realized that the boy had not much practice in handling money, and we were assuming that he had now 'learnt his lesson'. We would lend him a couple of pounds to be repaid in weekly instalments of ten shillings a week, with an assurance that if he tried it again he would get a dusty answer. I never lost a penny over transactions of this kind, and only very rarely indeed did anyone even get behind with his repayments. Indeed, as often as not I forgot to ask for them, and would be reminded by the boy producing an extra ten shillings with his £3 5s od.

Here perhaps it is appropriate to refer to another inconsistency. In spite of what was said above about a boy's money being entirely at his own disposal, there was an exception to this for those few boys who were not paying the full £3 5s od a week for their board and lodging. To them the line would be:

'Insofar as you are not paying the full fixed charge for "rent", we are in effect giving you so much a week. This we do because your wages are so low, and we do not want you to be deprived of the necessities of life such as clothes. It is my duty to the people providing that money to see that it is used for the purposes for which it was provided. I am not interfering with your earnings but I am supervising the use of something that has been added to them.'

The boy would then be required to place ten shillings a week in a personal clothing fund in my keeping. From this fund he could draw without let or hindrance at any time, subject only to the proviso that he must produce a receipt proving that it had been spent on clothes. As was made clear above, this applied only to very few boys. It was, in the main, resented by the few boys to whom it was applied, and several were known to insist on paying the full 'rent' although they need not, rather than be required to save in this way.

About two-thirds of the boys rapidly learned how to handle
their money, and a few arrived with a mature attitude already fully
developed. Of the remainder, about half learned this important lesson
only after much tribulation and a great deal of encouragement; the
other half consisted of the pathological cases: the incorrigibly spendthrift and the incorrigibly stingy. It amused me from time to time to put
them at each other's service. If I found a spendthrift about to commit
himself to some expensive hire-purchase scheme, I would say to him,
'Why don't you ask Robert to lend it to you? He's got oodles of cash,
and he'd only charge you 5 per cent instead of the 10 per cent or 15 per
cent these people want.' Robert was delighted to earn 5 per cent on his
investment, the debt was kept in the family, and its repayment could
be informally supervised. It was also public knowledge within the
hostel, and a certain amount of hostile opinion would be expressed
about the stinginess of the one and the recklessness of the other, which
would do neither of them any harm, and might indeed do them good.

This raises the vexed question of buying on the never never. This
is difficult for me because I had a puritan white-collar-working-class
upbringing, and have never been able entirely to shake off the conviction that to acquire something before you have paid for it is not
only improvident and reckless; it is also sinful. Of course a reputable
firm will not give credit to a minor unless he has a guarantor, and
I have once or twice had the pleasure of telling representatives of less
reputable firms that they knew perfectly well they could not enforce
collection from a minor, and that as I also knew this they need not call
any more. But at Reynolds House we had no trouble of that kind,
largely because we kept our debts in the family. Boys would come to
ask me to guarantee a credit purchase, and it was a difficult decision to
make. In the early days I just made it understood that this was something I never did, but in time reason triumphed over my puritan
upbringing. Joe wanted to buy a motor bike. He was earning good
money, and was a reliable payer. If he had had a father, a real father
that is, his father would have made it possible for him to get his bike,
as so many fathers do. His father might have paid for it himself, he
might have made a contribution towards the cost, he might have lent
some or all of the money, he might have guaranteed a hire purchase
agreement. I could not feel it to be right that Joe should be deprived
of his bike simply because he had also been deprived of a father. So
I told him that when he had saved up the deposit I would sign the
form and (at his request) go with him to make the purchase. I never
regretted this, even though Joe did make a fool of himself over that

bike in one way or another. Later I signed several more guarantees of one kind or another, though not unless I was sure the boy could afford what he was proposing to buy and could be relied on to pay regularly. I was never once called upon to pay, and only twice had to remind a boy who had missed a payment or two that it was my good name he was trifling with as well as his own. I believe some of my colleagues acted as guarantor in this way with similar results. Sometimes we lent money, even quite large sums. One such sum financed the purchase of a car. I also lent £20 for a second-hand drum set, which was paid with punctilious regularity at £1 a week. I used to make rather a noise about my personal integrity, my punctilio in money matters and so on, and I believe my debtors got some satisfaction from demonstrating that they were equally punctilious. I speak of my own money-lending activities because those are the ones I know about, but I fancy my colleagues lent more than I did. The boys tended to go to 'their' adult for this sort of thing. Mrs S., I know was very generous, and probably the only person who actually lost any money in this way – £2.

In fact the moneys paid by the boys made no difference to the hostel's income. Each boy was maintained by a local authority, and the moneys paid by the boys were offset against what was payable by the authority, and thus by the local ratepayer. The strategical reasons for minimizing this aspect in dealing with the residents were two: because it was felt necessary to enhance their feeling of independence, and to discourage any feeling that it did not matter whether, or how much, they paid.

CHAPTER SEVEN

LEISURE

Unclubbability is endemic among maladjusted young people, and the leisure occupation of the residents was perhaps the least satisfactory side of the hostel's life. But it may well be that in the free atmosphere that was provided, the residents took what they needed rather than what we thought might be good for them. This is something the emotionally disturbed very often do with great success if the opportunity is provided, and is one of the many reasons why a free libertarian atmosphere is preferable to a tightly structured directive one.

I am not implying that a busy social life is essential to happiness or stability, indeed there are many pursuits that can be followed in solitude. But there are few that are not enhanced by being shared, and the solitary life, to be satisfactory, demands greater inner resources than were at the disposal of most of the residents of Reynolds House. They came to the hostel from more or less closed communities in which they had lived for years, some of them for the greater part of their lives, and their leisure time activity had usually been catered for largely within that small community. When the boys reached Reynolds House our aim was to try to secure their integration into the larger community, and it was hoped that this might be done through the medium of their own interests. Consequently not much was done to cater for those interests within the hostel; instead a great effort was made to introduce them to people of like interests outside the hostel. It was a dismal failure. With the enthusiastic help and support of the borough youth officer, a very good friend of the hostel, boys were repeatedly introduced to youth clubs. The club leader, privily apprised of their difficulty in relating, would go out of his way to make them feel at home and to introduce them to other young people; but all to no end. The lad would go to the club for a week or two and then stop. Even those few, not more than a half a dozen in the five years, who retained membership of a club for more than two or three weeks, were never more than half-hearted in their enthusiasm and loyalty, and never seemed to acquire a real sense of belonging. Discussing this phenomenon among ourselves, we decided that perhaps our mistake had been to try to rush them into clubs too soon before they had acquired a feeling of security in their new home, so we tried postponing introduction to clubs until the boy seemed to have got roots down at the hostel. This met with no more success, and well-settled boys had no more use for youth clubs than new boys.

So much for youth clubs. The efforts to introduce boys to organizations catering for specific interests or talents met with no better success. My colleagues and I got in touch with a number of societies and organizations because some boy was interested in their speciality, all to no end. I never tried to push any boy into church, but I did make contact with the local clergy of various denominations, none of whom seemed interested. No boy was ever involved in any kind of art group, though several were quite 'arty', nor into any dramatic society or anything of that kind. Interest was often expressed, but they always jibbed at joining an organization. In the whole five years only one boy joined a football club, for which he played regularly for a couple of seasons. One boy attached himself to a small cine-club, but after a couple of months joined the Navy, so that was the end of that. Several boys thought they had interests which, however, they then found to be somehow more appropriate to their old life than their new one. Fishing was one of these, model-making another. Joe was the only boy who fished with regularity, though several expressed great interest, and had fished before, and even bought expensive equipment with their new wealth but they caused no concern to the fish. Two boys had guitars on which they could play passably well for beginners, but neither ever joined a group. One boy bought a drum set but used it almost exclusively for amusing himself in the bedroom.

There is of course a possible reason for this determination (as it seemed) to stay at home, apart from the difficulty that most of them experienced with human relationships. Reynolds House was home-like and it provided for a large number of its residents their first experience of real, comfortable home life. Indeed it was more homelike than home in the sense that it was child-oriented, while the ordinary family home tends to be, quite naturally and properly, also adult-oriented. It was *their* home and not, except incidentally, the staff's. They could watch the TV programmes that appealed to them, and were not restricted to the programmes father wanted to see. Above all else, they could listen to their kind of music, tuned to that deafening volume which alone seems satisfactory to the young. So while they had this home, and they knew they only had it for a couple of years or so, they enjoyed it. Pop music and TV, the main interests of most of them, were freely available at all times and seasons, except insofar as the housemeeting might see fit to regulate their use. A few boys did from time to time visit discotheques of varying degrees of shadiness, but not very often.

In the winter evenings various table games of the Monopoly type had periods of popularity, as did chess, draughts and cards. Here again they displayed a well-known characteristic of the maladjusted child, they always wanted an adult to play with them. They did of course often play without an adult, but there was usually an attempt to get an adult into the game, and we all spent many evening hours at Rummy and Canasta and Monopoly and Careers, and at what seemed to me a most particularly tedious and boring game called Risk, concerned with world conquest by military power which was however quite fascinating to them. Whatever unconscious motives lay behind this need to have an adult playing, the presence of an adult in the game did at least tend to reduce the number of squabbles over it as the adult was always assumed to be umpire, and his view of the rights and wrongs of a situation was rarely questioned. I was less often involved in chess and draughts, because it seemed unwise to get oneself completely tied up with one boy for most of the evening, with the rest of the boys probably in another room. For a period there was a passion for playing cards for small stakes. This was killed not by being banned as morally reprehensible but because it became such an unutterable bore to the non-players. The gamblers would sit with their heads over the table, totally engrossed in their cards and little heaps of coppers, so that it was impossible to get a civil word out of them, or ever get the use of the table for any other purpose. My attempts to ridicule them out of it met with only limited success; it was the housemeeting that finally put a stop to it.

We spent hundreds of man-hours watching violent rubbish on the TV, as the set was switched from channel to channel to ensure getting the maximum amount of violence. I cannot believe that all this TV violence, verbal and physical, is going to be without its effect on our social life. Watching it, as they do hour after hour and night after night, I do not see how these young people can avoid making the assumption that what goes on there with such monotonous regularity, is a reflection of ordinary life as it is lived: life in which business moguls habitually speak to each other in tones of insufferable offensiveness; husbands and wives do nothing but quarrel together and fornicate apart. It is quite customary and acceptable if someone says something you do not like, to smash your fist into his nose or your knee into his groin; and shooting is going on all the time everywhere. We were occasionally allowed to see something worth watching; not because we asked for it but because fortunately not all the boys wanted to watch rubbish all the time, and occasionally interesting and perhaps even fruitful discussions would follow a TV documentary. One young man, however, had the scarifying experience of seeing his mother in a documentary about women in prison.

The one other important interest of the residents was of course auto-mechanics. Boys would buy old motor-cycles for five pounds or so, or an old car for not much more, and would then spend far more happy hours tinkering with them than they ever spent riding or driving them. One summer in particular there were no fewer than seven vehicles, two of them four-wheelers. The deputy Warden would walk round the front and back yards and side-area – all littered with vehicles in varying stages of *déshabille*, advising each boy in turn on the next step to take in whatever operation he was carrying out, like a garage foreman supervising his fitters. He is an unusual man in the sense that although his interests are primarily intellectual, he is also remarkably well-informed and competent over practical affairs. He is a superb handyman, and the odd bits of damage about the place, or pieces of machinery that went wrong, would be promptly put in order by him in the most efficient and workman-like way. But what was of even more value was that he was knowledgeable about so many of the things in which the boys were interested. He knew all about electronics, and could say what was wrong (and often put it right) when a radio was out of order; he even helped a boy to construct a competent radio receiver in, if I remember rightly, a matchbox. He is skilled in working with wood and metal, and knows all about the internal combustion engine. If a boy's fishing rod got stuck or his airgun was out of order, Ron would show him how to put it right. It can be imagined how valuable an asset such a man was in such a place.

Then of course there were girls. These would be picked up in cafés or cinemas or in the street, and some of them seemed very pleasant and well-conducted young women. When I was an adolescent, there were two kinds of girl, those you picked up and those you had been introduced to, and only the second kind were taken home or intro-duced to parents; the other kind one did not even admit knowing. Generally speaking, the girl one picked up was, as the saying goes, 'Not much class'. All that is gone, and what a splendid thing it is! Even now a girl does not admit she has been picked up, but it is easy now to scratch an acquaintance so that there is very little difference. So the girls who were picked up (in whatever sense) by our boys were often very nice. Some of them of course were not, but a large proportion were. The boys would bring them into the house but often seemed quite at a loss about how to entertain them. A significant and remarkable symptom of their hesitancy in the whole matter of girl-friends was their quite astonishing willingness to accept advice about a girl's suitability. On one occasion a group of girls was brought into the house and, following a quite frequent practice, left in the common room watching television while their young hosts went into the dining room for Sunday high tea. I had seen these girls, of course, and thought very little of them. Without the slightest hope that my words would be in the least regarded, I said at large over the tea-table, 'I don't think much of that lot. I should think you'd better get rid of them. Surely you can find something better than *that*!' By the time I had finished tea and washed-up, they were gone. On several occasions after boys had brought girlfriends to me for inspection, I would say 'Huh, don't think much of *that*', or 'Not your sort, dear boy. Find something better', and she would be dropped. Just like that. This astonished me, and I record it not as a tribute to my influence, but as an indication of the complete lack of confidence in this matter among the boys. I think they would have taken less notice of my views on this subject if my general attitude had been an authoritarian one and if I had expressed my views as orders or instructions rather than as take-it-or-leave-it opinions. It is worth remembering, too, that only two of all the boys who came to us had been to co-educational schools, and some of them had been for the greater part of their lives in a one-sex environment. The two boys who had been at co-educational schools showed noticeably more aplomb than the others in their dealings with girls, though the most distinguished hunter of girls, it must be said, came from a boys' school. The fact that he chased girls interminably and had a measure of success in his girl-hunting does not mean that he knew what to do with them, except in one respect, or how to treat them when he had got them. However, we did not really have many girls about the place, and sometimes months would pass without a girl crossing the threshold, again one presumes because of this endemic difficulty over relationships. Three or four boys in the five years had a steady girlfriend, and two were engaged to be married, one at the age of sixteen and one at the age of seventeen.

Of parties there were very few, because we would not organize them. It was my view that if they wanted a party they should organize it. After all, they knew far better than an old fogey like myself what they wanted, and of course we were willing to give them any help they needed. From time to time parties were proposed at the housemeeting but rarely indeed did they come to anything. The chief problem was that they would not invite people, or the people they did invite failed to turn up. I remember one occasion when my wife at the request of the housemeeting, made elaborate catering arrangements, and not a soul turned up. The next night, Henry went out and brought back about fifteen or twenty young people, very pleasant if not indeed 'superior' young people, art students and the like, and an impromptu party was held, but without the elaborate catering arrangements of the night before. Alcohol was always a problem on these occasions. To hear them talking when a projected party was being discussed it seemed that their whole idea of fun at a party was to drink too much. Most of them of course were below the statutory age for drinking in pubs, though that did not prevent some of them from doing it from time to time, but we felt we had a duty to provide a little education in the right use of liquor so far as we could. So there would be a few bottles of brown ale available at parties, and some sherry perhaps, or a bowl of punch. Our idea was that in a good family the children would drink as much as their parents gave them, but it was difficult to restrict the boys to that. One clever lad brought in a miniature bottle of Vodka and poured it in his girlfriend's glass of beer with the result that she was horribly sick. But such episodes were very rare and we never had any drunkenness at a party. On the rare occasions when parties did take place the main problem about which we worried was that of uninvited guests. This could be a real problem in the neighbourhood. Word would go round the town that a party was being held at such a place, and crowds of young people, often carrying bottles (and often with the contents of several already inside them) would turn up and sweep through the place like a tornado. But in this, as in so many things, our fears were unfounded. I braced myself to do battle at the door, but it was never necessary, the residents took care of that themselves, and we never had an unwanted guest.

One party we did arrange every year was the Christmas Day party. I always dreaded Christmas, which was a very difficult time for our young men, partly because of their adolescent state and partly because of their homelessness. As children, which adolescents still are, they looked forward to Christmas with vague expectations of a kind of magical happiness, when something quite exceptional and out of this world would take place, and of course the reality was always disappointing. They looked forward to they knew not what, and the nearer the day approached, the greater were their fears that their hopes would not be realized. As adults, which adolescents also are, they looked forward to Christmas, I regret to say, as a time of drunken roistering and ribaldry, and of course they did not get that either. Then again, Christmas is pre-eminently the festival of the home, and although we did our best, Reynolds House was not really home.

So at Christmas the boys were apt to be sad without exactly knowing why, very much on edge, seeking they knew not what, but quite sure that what was provided was not that thing. After the first year, when we realized how child-like was one aspect of their feelings about this festival, my wife very wisely insisted that we should, in some ways, treat them as children, and fill their stockings. It was charming and pathetic to see how much this was enjoyed and appreciated, though the enjoyment and appreciation were visible only to him who had eyes to see. There was a Christmas tree, and an enormous exchanging of presents: adults to each other and to residents, residents to adults, but never, so far as I could ever see, residents to each other. There was the usual excessive eating and drinking, and in the evening, until the small hours, a domestic party in our flat. For the last three years the tree and its decorations and the wine for dinner were all provided by an 'old boy' who lived near by.

The party consisted of the usual old-fashioned party games. Rarely did such a party take place without one or two sad and wrought up young men saying they were not coming, and affecting to go out or sit below watching TV, but they usually turned up sooner or later. Equally rare was it for the party to reach its end without someone rushing out in a paddy because he claimed not to be 'out', or because someone had quite innocently laughed at him. But I am sure, nevertheless, that they were appreciated, and often in the ensuing weeks some of these professedly hard-boiled young men would demand that we played the party games, demands which I tended to resist so as to retain their magical Christmas quality.

Although, then, I always dreaded the approach of Christmas, my worst fears were never realized, and indeed our last Christmas passed off without even a minor hitch. Of course what I really dreaded was not the things that might happen but the underlying current of sadness and disappointment which I knew I could really do nothing to allay. There is no remedy for bereavement, and these boys were bereft of some of the fundamental necessities of satisfactory human existence.

There was another respect in which the adults really went to town in an effort to organize something for the residents. High days and odd holidays we expected the housemeeting to do something about, and usually, though not without a little prodding, they managed to arrange something or other. Annual holidays were another matter, and these the adults did try to organize. We made no attempt to take them all to camp or to organize any kind of group holiday. Holidays we saw not only as an opportunity to see new places, but also, what was of prime importance to our young men, to meet new people. But they almost defeated us. For most of them the idea of going alone (or even with a friend) to a strange place among strange people was something to be dreaded, and much as they may have longed for the excitement of a foreign holiday with other young people, their basic insecurity and fear of the unknown very often prevented them from taking the opportunities that were offered.

With the generous financial help of the Chase Charity, a scheme was arranged which made it possible for every boy to have, within certain limits, the holiday of his choice. Participants paid weekly into a holiday fund at the rate of 1s (later 1s 3d) in the pound of their 'free'-money, i.e. the money they had left when they had paid for their board and lodging. This meant an average payment of about 2s 6d a week for nine or ten months of the year. They were then invited to choose their holiday from a variety placed before them in a made-up brochure compiled with cuttings from the advertising booklets of organizations or companies catering specifically for young people. All kinds of exciting holidays were available in all parts of Europe and the British Isles, but rarely was it possible, even at so small a cost, to induce more than half the boys to go away. All, or nearly all, would pay into the fund, but would begin to drop out, sacrificing all they had paid in, for it was clearly understood from the beginning that there would be no repayments as the holiday season drew near. All manner of excuses were presented, few of them having much basis in reality. Some would drop out after deposits had been paid, some at the very last minute after reservations had been completed. The only year that most of the boys actually went away was 1968 and that was because my colleague, the sub-warden, defeating, in a way, the purpose of the project, offered to go with a party if a party could be arranged. Even so, three of his original party of six dropped out, though one of them was replaced at the last minute.

There were always one or two who suffered less from these fears, and over the years boys went as far afield as Istanbul (on a 'minitrek'), Yugoslavia (to a work camp), Holland, Germany, Switzerland, Paris, Ireland (cycling), and Wales (canoe-camping), apart from the above party which went to the Austrian Tyrol.

To return to the everyday life of Bromley, drugs never became a problem. There was the odd pep-pill acquired at a discotheque, and one boy got some reefers at a pub, but was picked up by the police before he had even tried them. He asked me what I thought they would do. I said that in view of his unblemished character, and the kind of things I should say about him at the court, the chances were that he would be given a conditional discharge. He then told the probation officer that if the court did their duty they would give him a conditional discharge. The probation officer (rather unkindly I think) passed on this information to the court. They, intending it appears to do that very thing, felt that they could hardly take their instructions from the defendant, so they fined him £5.

It is probably true to say that in the informal, relaxed and intimate atmosphere of the house, the staff very quickly became aware of any undesirable practice, current or imminent. Occasionally a boy would experiment with alcohol, and perhaps discover one day to his surprise that he had taken more than he could carry. But this too was rare.

For those who have left school, education is in the nature of a leisure time activity, and some boys went to evening classes, usually with the strictly utilitarian aim of accumulating GCEs in order to improve their prospects at work. Only four were ever serious students in this way, and three of them did acquire 'O' levels. One has since returned to full-time education at a college of further education, and is at present seeking a university place. Two or three others took non-examination subjects like physical training and motor-cycle maintenance, and that was the extent of evening school activities.

In one respect we departed from the policy of not laying on activities in the hostel. My wife had been by profession an art therapist, and she provided from time to time supervised opportunities for painting and drawing. This facility was appreciated and used, but her preoccupation with domestic affairs severely restricted the time she was able to give to it. There were usually two or three boys who were specially interested in art, and these she was able to encourage individually to pursue their interest. A good deal of painting was done in this way, including two murals. One of these was so expressive of the depressed condition of the artist, that after he had left the opportunity of spring-cleaning was taken to remove it. The other still decorates the wall of the half-landing.

In spite, however, of the dissatisfaction felt by the adults with the leisure activities of the residents, and perhaps our standards were too high, it is not thought that they were particularly dissatisfied themselves; though they did from time to time complain of boredom as all adolescents do.

It was during their leisure hours that our neighbours were apt to become aware of the boys. Our 'neighbour' on one side was a large and superior garage which had along its frontage a row of imposing standard lamps, hardly distinguishable from street lighting. The end lamp was almost opposite our side area, and proved one day to be too tempting a target for certain marksmen with an airgun. I knew nothing of this, and if the garage people knew, they said no word but simply had the damage repaired at some considerable cost. A little while later exactly the same thing happened again. The third time it happened even our kind and long-suffering neighbours felt that they had had enough, and one of the directors came to see me. He did not pick up his telephone and bellow down it, he came to see me. He was quite embarrassingly apologetic, and one would have thought that I was the wronged party and he the offender. He realized what a difficult task I had, he knew that we could not expect perfect behaviour from boys who had suffered the early experiences to which some of our boys had been subjected, the last thing in the world he wanted to be was a complaining neighbour. When I found an opportunity to express *my* regrets, I asked him to let me have a bill. Oh no, he would not think of that. If I could just try to persuade the airgun owner to find some other target in the future he would be perfectly satisfied. But I insisted. I said I wanted the bill, and I assured him that it would not be paid by me nor by my employers. At last he consented and in due course I received a bill for four or five pounds, only the cost of the last outrage, not the first two. The following Sunday I presented this bill to the housemeeting, who identified the culprits in a matter of minutes, and arranged for the bill to be paid.

Not all our neighbours went to quite that degree of forbearing charity, but they nearly all approached it in varying degrees. Behind the garage was the Bromley Cricket Club, and I can quite understand the fury of the groundsman and players when they found a puppy from the hostel digging great holes in their immaculate 'table'. Unfortunately, they made the mistake of merely swearing indiscriminately at such of the residents as they happened to see instead of asking for me, with the result that I did not realize how serious the matter was until I got a letter from their solicitor. We got rid of the pup which was in fact almost as much a trespasser on our land as he was on theirs.

I urged all seven of our neighbours to let me know if the boys ever impinged on their privacy, made too much commotion, or annoyed them in any way. One old gentleman who lived on the side street, and whose garden marched with ours, from time to time did so, but he also called in from time to time with periodicals for the quiet room. His complaints usually had some justification, but on one occasion I thought they had not and told him so. He stormed from the house threatening all manner of drastic action against us. About an hour later he telephoned and said, 'I've been thinking about what you said, Mr Wills. You were quite right. I'm sorry'. He was a gentleman. Where he is now he is neighbour to the Cherubim and Seraphim, who, as we all know, continually do cry! I wonder what he makes of that.

That was the extent of our trouble with the neighbours, who were kind, friendly, forbearing, understanding. But this happy state of affairs did not come about entirely by chance, and in fact we went to great lengths to secure their goodwill. As soon as we were ready to receive our first resident we had an open day where sherry was dispensed and the work of the hostel described. To this we invited all the immediate neighbours and certain more distant neighbours who were known for their public spirit and interest in social problems. In addition, anyone else who might conceivably be interested was invited: social workers, ministers, magistrates, probation officers, police. At the official opening a couple of months later a wider range of public-spirited people was invited, and social workers and local government officers from further afield who might one day want to send a boy to the hostel.

There is no doubt that these functions paid dividends. Whenever people outside, neighbours, magistrates, social workers, came into contact with residents there was at least a very good chance that the name of the hostel would mean something to them, that they would have at least some idea of the kind of boy they were dealing with and would be ready to adopt an understanding and sympathetic attitude to them.

We took great pains, too, to avoid giving offence to the neighbours, even though it sometimes meant giving offence to the residents who thought the lengths I went to try to stop them from upsetting the people around us were crazy. I told them, however, that it was all very well for them, but when somebody came round to blow his top, it was I, not they who had to suffer the wrath. It is true that the boys raised the volume of their radios and record players to the excruciating pitch that satisfied them, but at such times I insisted on all windows facing other people's houses being tightly closed. The large lawn was used only for sitting about on and never as a games park. I even objected to boys sitting there on a sunny Sunday afternoon with the radio quietly playing, much to their indignation. (But of course if it was really quiet I could always fail to hear it if I wanted to.) Boys who wanted to rev. up their motor bike engines in the exasperating way that they have were begged and implored to restrict such exercises to the side or front of the house, where the neighbours would not hear. I suffered a good deal of odium from the boys over this sort of thing, and had the greatest possible difficulty in convincing them that no person has any right to inflict his particular kind of noise on other people. In this I was much helped by our neighbours, who were as meticulous as I tried to be in keeping themselves to themselves, and practising that rule about not interfering with other people's liberties which I tried so hard to inculcate in our boys.

Some of the boys of course appear from time to time at the magistrates court, sometimes for stupid childish pranks, such as telephoning Scotland Yard to say that some young slobs were interfering with the public call box. It seemed so successful the first time that they tried it again, and when they came out of the booth a couple of policemen were waiting for them. Sometimes they appeared for traffic offences, and occasionally on more serious charges. The first time I went to Bromley Court with some of our young men I was so much impressed with the way the court was conducted, with the compassionate and understanding way in which they dealt with the offenders, not only ours, but others that I heard while I was waiting, that I felt impelled to write to the Chairman and tell him this. I got to know the magistrates better as time went on, partly as a result of my appearances at court with boys, partly as the first lay member of the probation and aftercare committee and the local probation case committee. I never had occasion to amend the opinion formed on that first occasion. Bromley was very fortunate in its bench of magistrates, and so were our boys though I'm not sure how far they realized it.

The interest of the public in the work of the hostel had one serious drawback, there were too many visitors. As the hostel had been conceived as a pilot project which it was hoped others might copy, we were bound to feel that such visits should be encouraged, but they were a great burden and we usually tried to arrange for them to take place during the middle of the day when fewest boys were likely to be about. But there were always some boys around, and they tended to resent it. One or two felt so strongly about it that they could not conceal their hostility ('Wot the bloody ell do *you* want 'ere then?'), but fortunately the visitors were very understanding. One boy, who used to come home to lunch, became extremely heated at the behaviour of the grocer's representative. This gentleman used to call once a week to receive the grocery order, and it happens that he usually called about lunch time. Being a kind and thoughtful man, and knowing that we were probably at lunch, if he happened to find the front door open he would walk in and wait in the kitchen until he was discovered there. This thoughtful act aroused the greatest fury in poor Henry, who would want to know by what right that bleed'n sod was walking into *our* house as if it belonged to him. There is no doubt that this resentment of visitors was to some extent the measure of the degree to which the residents felt the hostel to be their home, and the problem has no easy solution.

CHAPTER EIGHT

ADOLESCENCE AND SEPARATION

My wife and I took on the job when I was sixty, knowing that I should have to retire at sixty-five. It was, therefore, possible for us calmly and dispassionately to observe at our leisure the problems raised by the departure of the parent figures, and to try to deal with them as, if not indeed before, they arose. That has never been possible for me before. For the first time therefore I am in a position to say something about what some call separation anxiety. the symptoms of which form a significant part of many of the well-known symptoms of adolescence; for adolescence is the period of the second great separation in our lives.

The first great separation of course was parturition, and infancy is very much akin to adolescence. At birth we are wrenched from the perfect comfort, warmth and security of the womb, to the big, buzzing confusion of this world, and it must be a terrifying experience, ameliorated though it is by the constant care and solicitude, the fussing, smiling and crooning, of a doting mother. If a child is denied that amelioration, even for a matter of weeks, the experience is liable to leave its mark, and the child may find himself in time in a school for maladjusted children, an approved school, or a psychiatric hospital.

We obliterate infancy from our memory and I often think the same thing happens with adolescence, when I hear some middle-aged people talking about 'young people nowadays'. Certainly we are apt to forget a great deal of it. It is, among other things, a period of great distress and tension, of discomfort, strain and worry. Worry, to be sure, about many things which we shall later regard as trivial, but which then had all the emotional content of a matter of life and death. We may remember the thrill and rapture of first love, but we forget the acute distress about what she might think of our adolescent pimples, or the despair we felt because the particular shirt we wanted to wear to meet her was not back from the wash. It is a period of extremes, rapture and despair, despair and rapture, and those of us who survive it tend to remember the rapture but forget the despair, when we talk about youth being the happiest time of our lives.

Even, however, if we blot out only some instead of all this experience, adolescence is very much like infancy. To the infant all is new and compared with prenatal existence much of it must be unpleasant. To this confusing and uncomfortable world the infant has to learn to adjust. He has to learn how to distinguish between self and not-self, then how to relate to the not-self, how to communicate, which things bring pleasure and which pain, and how to gain the one and avoid the other. By the time he goes to school he has more or less learned all that, but only at a certain level. He has learned how to adjust as a child among children in a world of adults. He has adjusted to the childhood state, and for the next six or eight years nothing more is demanded of him and he demands nothing more for himself. It is a modified womb in which he now lives in which he retains strong links with the mother, and it is possible that, if he is in a good and loving home, he is during this period happy.

But when childhood begins to change to adulthood, everything is to do again. During that period of childhood which the Freudians call the latency period any changes that take place are changes of degree rather than of kind; he becomes taller and heavier, he adds to the sum of his factual knowledge. Now, as his happy, secure latency period draws to its end, he begins to make changes in kind. He has to begin to make adjustments to a new kind of life that is almost as unknown as the new life he entered at birth. Of course, he has seen adults, has formed conceptions of 'good' and 'bad' adults, has talked vaguely from time to time about 'when I am grown up', but all that was rather in the nature of fantasy than of real apprehension of what it means to be grown up. Now he sees the grown-up state actually approaching, sees it as something to be grappled with and understood, and indeed, he hopes, enjoyed, but no longer as something to dream about. The adjustments he made as a child are no longer adequate, any more than the prenatal adjustments he made in the womb are adequate after birth. He has now to adjust as a man among men, to acquire an adult attitude to life, adult modes of behaviour, learn how to cope with the sex thing that now looms up; in a real sense much of it is as new and as frightening as all the things the new-born infant had to adjust to and learn about.

Most young people have the appearance of entering this period with eagerness and confidence, and seem to be all too eager to assume complete adulthood almost overnight, but there is good reason to suppose that they are also deeply apprehensive, frightened, sad and resentful. In fact the young person's attitude to growing up is acutely and distressingly ambivalent. He welcomes the freedom, he welcomes the sexual adventure, he welcomes the relative affluence of adulthood. But at the same time, though he is unlikely to admit this or indeed to be fully aware of it, he dreads the responsibilities that adulthood brings and resents the loss of his secure, carefree childhood. He welcomes the escape from parental tutelage, and often seems eager to break loose too soon; but at the same time he is mourning what is in effect a kind of death to his parents. He sees escape from his parents not only as desirable, but also as inevitable, and dreads the end of his dependence on them, the end of the security he enjoyed as a child. His attitude to everything is therefore influenced by two contradictory urges: the urge to grow up, and the wish to retain the love, dependence and security of childhood, the urge to escape from his parents and the urge to retain them. Such acute ambivalence is not normal except during those few years. At any other time of life we should consider it pathological, and that is why I think of adolescence as a kind of sickness; that is why I say we are all maladjusted then.

When we come to consider the kind of young men who came to Reynolds House, or children in general in schools for maladjusted children, or children in care, we find this ambivalence intensified. In many cases they have not enjoyed, as other children have, several years of serene, unclouded childhood, and just because their childhood was so unsatisfactory they are the more anxious to leave it behind and start a new life. But it is security, and the happiness of the latency period which enables us to put down roots, and to acquire enough strength and stability to face the pains and dangers of maturity. 'Our' children have not had that, so while they are the more eager to become adults, they are also more apprehensive of adulthood and less able to cope with it than children emerging from a secure and happy childhood. They, even more than 'normal' children, are in the position of the ranks of Tuscany when Horatius held the bridge:

> But those behind cried 'Forward!'
> And those before cried 'Back!'

His conscious self cries 'Forward', but his unconscious self cries 'Back'.

All this has much of practical value to those of us who are concerned in a practical day-to-day way with adolescents, and I think it means we should conduct ourselves in a manner very different from the traditional way of dealing with such young people. The traditional way has been to assume, perhaps rightly, that they are in too much of a hurry to grow up, and are apt to demand more freedom and independence than they are ready for. The response to this has been to resist the young person's demands, reluctantly granting always a little less than the adolescent seeks, so that there are continual fights and upsets, the youngster usually getting his own way in the end, but with little satisfaction just because it was given so reluctantly. If there is any truth in what I have been saying, however, we know that while he is demanding to go forward he is also very apprehensive about it and reluctant to leave the security of childhood. Can we not exploit this for our own benefit and peace of mind? I think we can if instead of giving him reluctantly less freedom than he demands we should give him more, in the confidence that he will soon find it too much for him and ask us to place limits on it. But when they say 'What's wrong with smoking reefers?', do I say, 'Nothing at all, dear boy, here's a hypodermic, try a little snow, it gives you more of a kick than hemp?' No, because I suspect that if we adopt the attitude I am proposing, some of those outrageous demands would never be made. Some of them at least are an excessive reaction against the curbs we put on the young, and if the curbs were less the reaction would be less. I suspect that in our unconscious resentment against their growing up (for we have unconscious resentments as well as they), we bar many things that we need not bar, we 'advise' against many things that we need not advise against, so that they no longer trust our advice, and assume that all our prohibitions arise from the same anti-youth attitude that our unconscious resentment begot. They may know nothing about unconscious resentment, but they do know something about the innate impulse of the older to say No, because they have had experience of it. There is a simple rule to govern this question of whether to say yes or no. It is this: When some young person says 'May I do so and so?' and you immediately feel that you do not want him to do it, do not rear up. Just say to yourself, 'If he makes one hell of a fuss, and goes on and on, and wheedles and argues and all the rest of it, is there the slightest possibility that I might in the end give in?' If there is the remotest chance that the answer to this question could possibly be Yes, then say 'Certainly, dear boy, of course, with the greatest of pleasure', and save yourself a great deal of trouble, both now and in the future.

For those of us who run homes or hostels for adolescents, the implication of what I have been saying is not that we should tell the young that they are free to do just as they like, but simply that we should have the very minimum of rules and regulations, and it is surprising when you start examining them, how many rules are unnecessary. There were many instances at Reynolds House of boys asking to have their freedom curbed, asking indirectly, as Jim did, or quite directly, as did Joe. He had spent several pounds on an air-gun which he soon found he was not mature enough to use wisely. When he found that the freedom of owning an air-gun was more than he could cope with, he came and asked me to 'look after it' for him, which I very gladly did. Do not expect gratitude for all this freedom. They will take it for granted, they will grouse and grumble, they will even complain about their lack of freedom, but all this is to be expected: it is all part of the sickness called adolescence.

The approach I have been suggesting has other important lessons for us apart from this departure from the traditional in our general attitude. In several ways it helps us to understand and to forgive some of the most perplexing and exasperating things about young people. Ambivalence or duality for example helps us to understand one of the most outstanding characteristics of adolescence, namely that it is not a smooth and gradual progression from childhood to maturity. Nothing of the sort, it is a rough and irregular series of hops, skips and jumps, some forward, some backward, some sideways, of which the sum total over a long period of time, if all goes well, is a forward tendency. But to those of us who are condemned to live with these exasperating people, it sometimes seems as if they take a step back into childhood for every step towards maturity. Whatever we do, we must never get annoyed or upset about this because it is all a perfectly normal part of the condition. One day they will be obeying the injunction of those behind, the conscious self, to go forward; the next they will be heeding the voice of those in front, the unconscious fears, to go back. Indeed it is probably safe to say the greater any given step towards maturity, the greater the likelihood of a little reversion to childishness, because the very fact of taking a leap forward into the unknown country of adulthood activates the fears and apprehensions about leaving childhood. There is no need to rebuke them and tell them scornfully not to be childish, they need to be childish sometimes. Joey gave a magnificent example of this process. He decided that he was in the wrong job, but he did not, as many of his fellow-residents did, just chuck up his job and start looking for another. He went into the thing very fully and arrived at a very mature conclusion. He decided to go in for a trade which for the first few weeks, if not indeed months, he would earn less than he was getting at present, but which in a few months' time would give him a higher wage, and in the fullness of time a good and well-paid trade. He worked all this out with no help from me, merely reporting to me what he was doing. And in time he got his increase in pay and felt justified in making a splash with it. He spent several pounds on a child's elaborate train set with which he played a whole afternoon like a nine-year-old – and we never saw it again.

There is another symptom of this condition which the approach I am proposing helps us to understand. The adolescent, even if he is not a maladjusted adolescent, has one thing in common with the maladjusted child, though the symptom may have a different origin in each case. One of the significant characteristics of the maladjusted child is that in a vague, half-conscious kind of way, he feels that there is something lacking in his life. Very often he does not know what it is, and if asked about it he would probably have not the slightest idea what one was talking about. But we know what it is, though he does not. A large number of maladjusted children have been deprived, or feel themselves to have been deprived, of the absolute unconditional affection of parents which we all need if we are to grow into stable and dependable adults. They do not know that this is what is missing, but are half aware, in an indeterminate kind of way, of a feeling of something lacking, of a gap to be filled. Sometimes they try to fill this gap by taking possession of physical objects that are not theirs, frequently from the very person whose love they covet, but the more common effect is a generalized discontent, a feeling that all is not as it should be, that things would be better somewhere else. Does not this ring a bell with any who work with adolescents? Is not this exactly how they seem to feel? Is not this exactly in line with what Dr Stanley Hall said in his book about adolescence many years ago 'It is the eternal illusion of youth that gives elsewhere a greater charm'? Nothing is right, nothing is good enough, everybody else is stupid. He is lacking something too but in his case it is not the love he should have had in the past so much as the love he will have in the future. He is looking for a mate, and though he may chase the girls whenever he is free to do so, he does not realize that this sense of something lacking and therefore everything being wrong is due to the fact that until he does find a permanent mate he remains an incomplete person. It is he himself who is not quite as he should and hopefully will be, but of course he does not know and cannot see that, so he thinks it is his environment that is wrong. In a house with every kind of amenity and amusement, including TV, radio, record player and a library, he will still tell you from time to time how bored he is, and how he wishes there was something to do in this dump. You may think up all manner of exciting and interesting things for him to do, but the chances are he will have none of them, and understandably, because none of them is this vital thing he really wants, he really needs, to make him a complete person. In a town full of cinemas, clubs, theatres and everything else he will say 'What a dead and alive hole this is, nothing to do here, how I wish I lived somewhere else'. There is nothing we can do about it. There is no harm in trying of course, and indeed I think we should keep on trying, because sometimes we can suggest something that clicks for a time or something which, while it evokes no response now, may appeal to him later. But the great thing to remember is that this discontent is all part of the condition.

There is one other sense in which what I said earlier helps us to understand the adolescent and thus, one hopes, be more understanding and tolerant in our attitude, as well as less pessimistic about the results of what we are trying to do for him. There is a sense in which we may think of the adolescent as mourning the loss of his parents, his parents whom he is 'losing' by growing up and becoming an adult himself. But added to this is another quite different feeling which is also there though the young person is not aware of it. This is that when they begin to 'lose' their parents in this way it may be the cause of a great deal of unconscious resentment, resentment against them for the mere fact that they are going to allow themselves to be lost. Perhaps it is resentment against the mere fact of growing up and thus losing the security and support of childhood, but I suspect they tend to canalize it by directing it against the source of all that comfort and security they are losing, the parents who provided it and whose loss they are at the same time mourning. This resentment, furthermore, will be directed against anyone who has any kind of parent-relationship, actual or surrogate. We have all suffered from irrational and totally unprovoked ill-temper, general disagreeableness amounting at times to hostility. This is not the generalized discontent of which I spoke earlier, but something much more positive and unpleasant, which causes the young person to behave as if he positively hates you. Sometimes this hateful, abusive attitude is explained as being due to the restrictions that in the nature of things adults sometimes have to place upon the activities of adolescents, but I believe that to be a superficial explanation. I believe we should get it just the same if we imposed no restrictions at all, because it is not rational, as that would be, but a totally irrational unconscious resentment about the whole business of growing up. Parents get it, but so do parent substitutes, and the probability is that they will get it in an intensified form because they will also be having directed at them, as it were on transfer, the normal resentment that children can be expected to feel against their own parents who have failed them. Once we understand this, and it is all part of the condition, we shall find it much easier to bear, we shall be much less likely to reply in kind, to be angry, to indulge in recriminations about the abuse and general lack of appreciation we suffer or to be hurt by it. Blessed is he that expecteth nothing, for he shall not be disappointed, and we must never expect from the adolescent gratitude or appreciation or praise for anything we do. We must never expect this, but because he is such a highly unpredictable mortal we shall most surprisingly get our little tit-bits of rewarb from time to time, and lovely it is when it comes, though often recognizadle only by the very percipient or knowing.

I was told once at Reynolds House of an incident which was the very epitome of adolescent ambivalence. The victim was our dear Mrs S., the deputy matron, and the resident concerned was the one I have called Horace. After eleven o'clock one night, as Mrs S. was trying to go to bed, Horace banged on her door. 'Are you there, darling?' he said. 'Can I come in for a little chat, darling?' Mrs S. really wanted to go to bed, but she knew that Horace depended on her a good deal so she told him to come in. 'Thanks, darling' said Horace and in he went. He had no sooner got in than he began to abuse Mrs S., about nothing specific, without any cause, with no discernible end in view. He continued to revile her for a quarter of an hour or so, then said, Well, I better be getting along I suppose, darling. Mustn't keep you up all night. Good night, darling', and off he went. Poor Horace. He wanted the love and attention of a mother, the desire to remain a child, but he wanted it in the most inconvenient possible way, thus expressing the resentment he felt not only, as a maladjusted child, against his own inadequate mother, but also against Mrs S. for not being his real mother, and against the fact that he is rapidly growing up and will have to abandon the mother-child relationship before long. He called her darling because he loved her and wanted to retain her love. He reviled and abused her partly again in order to express his resentment, partly perhaps in order to convince himself that though he may be losing her, he was not after all losing much. But that was more than he could believe, and terrified of having lost her love by his abuse he ends by calling her darling again. Mrs S. fortunately is what we some-times call a natural, she knew how to respond without necessarily thinking out the reasons for it. She knew, as it were instinctively, that the very fact Horace felt this resentment and hostility meant that in the insecurity which gave rise to it he needed all her love. all her care and above all, all her tolerance. She listened not to the words he uttered, but to the need that gave rise to them, and it was to that alone she responded.

This leads on to the distress and anxiety that may arise in young people in residential establishments when staff leave, and especially when parent-figures leave. If adolescence is itself a kind of anxiety state, the anxiety being connected (among other things) with the impending separation from parents, and the loss of dependency that comes with adulthood, then we might expect the symptoms of separation anxiety to be much akin to the general symptoms of adolescence. And so in fact they prove to be. The condition of maladjustment often has its origin in early separation from parents; thus it is not surprising that some of the symptoms we associate with maladjustment are similar to those we associate with that gradual process of separation which we call adolescence. For the same reason we cannot be surprised if the child or young person undergoing separation from a key staff figure displays those same evidences of maladjustment. Indeed he is for the time being maladjusted, because that to which he was adjusted is being wrenched away from him.

Both these phenomena were to be seen at Reynolds House during our last year, when it has to be borne in mind not only that my wife and I were due to retire, but also that our colleague Mrs S. was due to retire a few months later. It is significant that during our first year we had no fewer than seven court appearances but as the residents established relationships with the staff, as they began to adopt us as parent-figures and became more secure, the number of court appearances dropped rapidly away to none in our fourth year. In the fifth year, however, the number of court appearances leapt suddenly to eight, though five of those concerned one boy. In the same way, our first year produced no fewer than seven transients – boys who came and did not stay, but the ensuing four years produced only three, of which one was in the fifth year and was clearly connected with our departure.

It may seem from the foregoing that our efforts to counteract the possible effects of our impending departure met with very little success, and certainly we had hoped for more; but I was confident, and so was our psychiatrist, that without those efforts the degree of disturbance would have been much greater. The following is an account both of these measures and of the symptoms displayed by individual residents.

The principal thing, of course, was to be as open as possible as soon as possible, and to avoid no opportunity of talking frankly and openly about the departure that was impending; firstly, in order to bring it into the open, and secondly, in order to provide opportunities to reassure. Anyone who has been engaged for long in residential work will have met people who, when they are proposing to leave, say nothing to the children until the very last minute. They say that this avoids upsetting the children, and so it may while they are there. The fact that when they have gone the distress is all the greater, will be someone else's worry. But if we say nothing to the children they nevertheless become intuitively aware of the fact that something is in the wind, and may feel deeply betrayed by the fact that their adult is up to something concerning which he is not prepared to take them into his confidence. An open, planned departure is, I venture to think, far less worrying and disturbing than a furtive, secret one. We, as I have said, had five years' notice of our departure, and the residents had the same notice. We never hesitated to refer to the fact that by the end of 1968 we should be gone, but of course this meant very little in the early days because clearly the residents concerned would be going before us. I also took care to point out to prospective residents during the penultimate year that I should probably be gone before they. During the greater part of the final year by design we did not receive any new residents.

By the end of our penultimate year (1967) we had admitted residents most of whom could expect to be still at the hostel when we left, but it was not until 1968 arrived, the actual year of our departure, that we were conscious of underlying anxieties. These signs were in most cases slight indeed, and might not have been noticed if we had not been looking for them; they were so slight indeed that, except for the major ones I shall refer to later, they cannot now be recalled, and only collectively amounted to a ponderable phenomenon. Most of the major signs were exhibited by specific boys, each in his own way, but there was one major sign that was common to all, and that was that our departure was never referred to, even after we had begun to notice the minor signs mentioned above. It is security I am talking about, not love, and so far as love enters the picture at all it is our love for them that is at issue, not theirs for us. The fact that they felt we liked and cared for them was one of the things that contributed to their basic feeling of security, and it was the threat of its removal that led to insecurity and distress.

During the mass separations brought about by evacuation during the war, it was, I think, commonly accepted that by and large the children who talked about their parents and referred from time to time to the fact of separation were less a source of anxiety to their hostesses than those who never mentioned parents, seemed entirely to have forgotten them. We assumed the same process would be at work in our case and considered it to be of prime importance that the matter should be brought to the surface. We therefore missed no opportunity during the last eighteen months or so of bringing it to the surface and discussing all its implications. This was not done in any formal way, but informally as opportunity arose, over a cup of tea in the quiet room, by the kitchen sink and so on. By the early summer of 1968, residents had begun to raise the subject themselves, and we felt that progress was being made. Some of them were even beginning to express their anxieties openly. They did not of course say 'We have come to rely on you, you provide us with a sense of security which we fear we may lose when you go'. They said, the more stable of them who did not need to use the oblique methods to which I shall shortly refer, 'What will the next Warden and Matron be like? Will they continue the meeting? Will they be tolerant of our misdemeanours? Will they be familiar and friendly, or will they be distant and authoritarian? Will they be able to manage so and so? Will the hostel be run as it is now, or will it become like those other places?'

To all these questions we replied with much confidence that the way the hostel was run was not a personal idiosyncrasy of mine, but was the way the Committee wanted it to be run, that was why they had appointed me and obviously they would find somebody with similar ideas who would run it in a similar way. Of course there would be minor differences: he would be a pretty poor mutt if he wanted to follow his predecessor slavishly, but his basic attitude, his basic approach, would be like mine. We also answered some of the unspoken questions which may have been in their minds by saying that we were retiring not dying, that we should keep in touch, that visits to our house in the country (which some of them had already made) would become easier once we had no formal duties and were there all the time . . . and so on. Applicants for the posts were introduced to the boys when they came to look over the premises and, when they had gone, the residents' opinions informally sought. The person appointed was in fact the one to whom the residents had clearly warmed, the only one of whom they had said 'Let's hope *that* one is appointed'.

The person was a woman, and once the appointment was decided upon she was encouraged, as she lived fairly near, to visit the hostel frequently. By this means it was hoped that the less stable residents might perhaps begin to lean on the new prop before the old one was taken away.

Some boys were able to refer to coming events only obliquely, and often offensively like the adolescent who, among other feelings, resents the fact that adulthood will in a sense deprive him of his parents, and directs this resentment to his parents by means of the well-known hostility of the teenager. So residents who had been reasonably friendly became at times uncharacteristically hostile. Sometimes they expressed their anxiety about the future in an offensive and 'inverted' kind of way such as, 'Perhaps we'll be able to have a bit of freedom for a change when the new Warden comes', which really meant, 'I fear the next Warden may impose a lot of the kind of petty restrictions which so far we have managed without'. Or, conversely, 'I'll be glad when the new Warden comes; I don't suppose she'll try to stop us staying up all night at the discotheque'. This was a particularly shady discotheque which I did try to keep them away from for very good reasons. This almost certainly meant, 'I hope the new Warden will be solid enough to help me to avoid the things I'm not quite strong enough to avoid on my own'. Or, 'For Chrissake mind your own bloody business, I hope to God the next Warden won't be for ever poking his nose in other people's business', this, after a perfectly casual and natural enquiry of the kind that anyone might make of anyone, such as 'Was it a good picture?', and undoubtedly meant, 'I hope the new Warden will be someone with whom we can with confidence discuss our intimate personal affairs'.

It may be thought that I am making a very speculative interpretation of these casual pieces of abuse. But there is some significance in the fact that while, of course, they had occurred from time to time in the past, they occurred now with much greater frequency, and often brought in the new Warden, who was a kind of symbol of their anxiety, and of the resentment they were expressing.

Among the most disturbed and apprehensive was Ronald. He had had a most unhappy and chaotic history, and although he had been for seven years in schools for maladjusted children he had never been happy there, nor in the children's home where he spent his holidays. A pathetic, unstable youth with all the classic symptoms of emotional deprivation, he came to the hostel about a year before we were due to retire. Although, in the circumstances we did nothing to encourage it, Ronald, somewhat to our distress, began to adopt my wife and me as parent figures. After a lifetime of encouraging such approaches as these, I suppose it had become almost second nature, and I was probably not as discouraging as I ought to have been. Ronald leaned on us, confided in us, and was clearly for the first time in his life enjoying some small measure of the kind of security that makes happiness possible. Of course he had his bad days, he was very unstable, but he was now for the first time in the kind of soil that suited him, and in which growth was possible. Ronald, stupid and unappreciative as he sometimes seemed, was undoubtedly aware of this, and was one of those who, in the spring preceding our autumn departure got himself involved in a burglary. Ronald, though an almost compulsive sneak-thief, had never done anything of this kind before, and this was his first appearance before the magistrates. He also became more and more hostile and abusive to me. Sometimes he would reply to my most harmless and casual observations with a storm of abuse. One mealtime (he usually sat quite close to me), I made some remark which might possibly have been interpreted as being faintly critical. Ronald rose up in a fierce but not uncontrolled rage. With great venom he leaned towards me and told me that I was a certain kind of bastard, that he had never liked me, that he had disliked me from the moment he met me, and still did, and always would, and would be glad when I was bloodywell gone. Is not this the kind of thing we get, though perhaps not quite so violently, from ordinary adolescents, directing against parents and parent figures the distress and resentment they feel at the fact they are soon to lose them, that they cannot become adult *and* continue dependence on parents? In the same way, Ronald was turning against me the resentment he felt that I was deserting him, casting him aside. A few hours later he was hanging, figuratively at any rate, round my wife's neck, talking to me as if we were the dearest of friends, saying how much he liked being at the hostel, what wonderful people we were. Then he was enjoying the present, earlier he had been dread-ing the future – two sides of the same medal. This is an exaggerated form of the typical behaviour of the adolescent, and the worker who cannot see the abuse and hostility of the young as the obverse of their love and dependency, will never get anywhere with them.

Living among unstable and often aggressive adolescents, it was no uncommon thing to be threatened with physical violence. One took little notice of it because one knew that it rarely meant 'I intend to assault you', but only, as a rule, 'At this moment, in my present violent rage, I wish that harm would come to you'. Of course the stupid or inexperienced worker can very easily turn this into an assault, especially if he himself is the kind of person who uses physical violence. I suffered violence when I was a very young worker, and used it myself, but during the last forty-five years I never suffered physical assault from an adolescent or adult until the last few months at Reynolds House when I was assaulted by Percy. It is true that he only pushed me, but he pushed me with some violence. I offered no resistance to his pushing, knowing that two or three pushes would bring me up against a wall and further pushing would be pointless. In fact I miscalculated and it was a door with glass panels that I came up against, with spectacular results. But that is by the way. The point is that this first attack in forty-five years was made by a boy who had until recently seemed quite devoted to me. Although Percy was reserved and pretty uncommunicative when in direct contact with me, he had praised me to others in a way that no resident ever had – and now he was assaulting me!

Poor Percy! His experience of life had been such as to make him afraid of any human relationship and it was not until he was about fourteen that he began to have, very tentatively, warm feelings towards his headmaster and his wife. They responded to his advances, but he was getting very near to school-leaving age. The headmaster in question was an old friend and colleague, that same Mr Penfold who had helped Tommy so much. He had worked with me in his formative years as a very young teacher, and had adopted, I was amused to learn from Percy, several of my mannerisms and verbal idiosyncracies. This made Percy feel that he was merely moving from one edition of Mr Penfold to another. It is true that he felt, rather than thought, of his leaving the school as a kind of rejection by the Penfolds, but he quickly established a good and useful relationship with me, a thing which the Penfolds had made possible. Percy was a very deeply disturbed boy and other influences were at work in his emotional life, including a very complicated and highly ambivalent relationship with his own father. But the fact that other influences may also have been at work does not lessen the significance of the particular chain of circumstances that I now relate. Percy had with difficulty learned tentatively to 'relate' to the Penfolds. They had seemed to reject him by sending him away, that is, by the normal and necessary process of school-leaving. However, that tentative beginning, and the special relationship I had with the Penfolds, made it possible for him to form another tentative relationship with me, and for the moment all seemed well. He came to us in the summer of 1967. As soon as 1968 arrived it was borne in upon Percy that I too was going to reject him by deserting him, and he had not yet acquired sufficient confidence in human beings to be able to believe that my interest in him would continue after I had left. This was so utterly daunting that all the good work of the Penfolds was undone and Percy erected a kind of steel shutter between himself and the world. The only feelings that could penetrate this shutter were feelings of intense hostility and resentment. Warmth was cut off, he did not any more believe in people, did not dare any more to make even tentative approaches to them. Deprived of warmth from outside, and the help to be derived from it, and terrified by the strength of his own hostility, he needed all the more some kind of security, and that he now sought. Deprived of the security that a suitable feeling relationship gives, he sought in desperation the security and protection of external control. He made a determined and eventually successful attempt to get himself taken into custodial care – where he now is.

Percy was a deeply disturbed boy in whom several baleful influences were at work. The fact remains, however, that if he had not felt I was deserting him, there was at least a sporting chance that he might gradually have acquired strength to counteract those other influences. Perhaps he still may, by strength provided from another source. But it is clear that his sense of rejection at a crucial moment in his life, just as he was beginning to acquire confidence in human beings, is something that it will be very difficult to overcome.

I have told Percy's story at some length to press home the point that constant changing from job to job by people engaged in this kind of work, whether in schools, homes or hostels, or to a lesser degree as child care officers, defeats the ends they seek to serve, and can bring distress immeasurable amounting even to ruined lives, to those they try to help. I repeat again the aphorism that Dr Donald Winnicott uttered to me many years ago. 'In this work the important thing is not so much to do it as to keep on doing it.'

CHAPTER NINE

AFTERCARE AND OUTCOME

Arthur was a student at a school of art, who had only been at the hostel five months when he was removed by his father, and taken to live with him. I kept in touch with him by occasional visits, and after a few months discovered that he had been expelled from the art school following some rowdyism in a pub. Poor Arthur was in a very depressed state, making no effort to earn a living, staying at home ostensibly working at his art, but actually getting very little on to canvas, and elaborating totally unrealistic plans for getting to college, for which he had no qualification. We discussed this situation at the case conference. My wife, who is an art therapist, had a high opinion of Arthur's talent, but this was not shared by the head of the school. It was felt at the case conference that we should try to get Arthur back to school, and I tried to see the head, but without success. He simply ignored my approaches, so at last in desperation I wrote to the chief education officer, explaining the circumstances and asking whether it was not possible for the expulsion to be changed to one year's suspension. This was eventually agreed to. Arthur duly returned to school and in the ensuing two years not only redeemed his artistic reputation in the eyes of the head, but gained enough 'A' levels to secure a college place. He has just finished his first year at art college.

I recount this as an admirable example of one of the aims of aftercare, which I see as having two entirely disparate aims. One, of which Arthur's is an example, is merely a matter of keeping an eye on things and taking such steps as may be necessary to help and advise the boy about his day-to-day affairs, occasionally putting in an oar, as I did here, if it seems necessary. Arthur had no great emotional dependency on the hostel, but he still needed our help over the day-to-day affairs of his life. The value of such help can hardly be over-estimated, and anyone who had seen Arthur three months after his expulsion, when there still seemed no hope of its revocation, would almost certainly have concluded that he was heading for a psychiatric hospital.

The other aim is quite a different one. It consists simply of the continuance of a relationship that was formed between the boy and the adult upon whom he was most dependent. One would have hoped that this might have been carried on by the school, but in fact it rarely was. It is now commonly accepted that in the majority of cases an essential element in the residential treatment of maladjusted children is the establishment of a warm affective relationship between the child and at least one of his environing adults. In many cases this will in due course make possible the repair of the damaged parent-child relationship which is so often present. In a few cases however, notably of the kind that are liable to come to Reynolds House, this adult-child relationship at the school has to be in some measure a substitute for the parental relationship. In such a case the worker must be prepared for a long period of greater or lesser emotional dependency on the part of the boy, though, once established, this does not necessarily mean being physically close at hand. It does mean, however, that when the boy is removed to another environment the worker must take great pains to assure the child of his continued interest, to make him feel that the worker is 'still there', though the presumption is that as stability and maturity increase, reliance on the worker will diminish. Obviously aftercare in this sense can be carried on only by the worker originally concerned with the child, though the other kind, the sort of operation that was carried on with Arthur, can be carried out by any competent social worker.

It may be thought that in practice we had very little aftercare to do because the boy was already in an aftercare situation in relation to his school, and he was already in the care of a social worker of one kind or another, a child care officer or a mental welfare officer. Alas, it did not work out like that. Very few schools carried out effective aftercare work with boys who came to Reynolds House, and, as we have seen, they tended to form very close ties with people at the hostel, so that it was necessary for us to undertake aftercare in the second sense, the continuance of a relationship. So far as the other kind was concerned, that too was found to be necessary, because while it is true that they were technically in the care of the local authority social worker, that care officially ceased as a rule at eighteen for boys in care. It is true that child care officers always assured the boy of their continued interest, and urged them to get in touch if they needed help, that is not the same thing at all as maintaining contact. Boys maintained by the health authority, as we have seen, had very little help indeed from mental welfare officers.

Aftercare, therefore, seemed to devolve upon us whether we wanted it or not. I have given an example of the social work kind of aftercare;

perhaps I should give one that illustrates the continuance of an affective tie.

Tommy, as we started with him in an earlier chapter, might be a good example. Though making good progress in general, and doing very well at work, he had a profound emotional dependence on the hostel, and was very apprehensive about leaving. We therefore kept him on long after his authority had abandoned responsibility for him, and ultimately eased him out with very great caution. Fortunately his place of work was quite near and when a bedsitter had been found for him he was encouraged to spend all his spare time at the hostel. For some months the only difference between him and the residents was that he slept elsewhere, and after two and a half years, he still looks in for at least a short time practically every day, and often spends his day off at the hostel. He has however matured a great deal, being enabled to do so because of the security provided by this relationship. He has been promoted to a very responsible position at work, and last year was sufficiently independent to take his holiday abroad.

Tom's and Arthur's are two success stories which without aftercare would have been failure stories. Eustace seemed for a very long time to have been a failure story, and although at this moment all seems well, it is too soon to be confident, though he had more aftercare in terms of time and trouble than any other resident. Like Tom's, his story is an example of the effort to maintain a relationship.

Eustace was an extremely difficult and unstable young man, sometimes frightened and unselfconfident in the extreme, at other times so wild and aggressive that his fellow residents were terrified of him. His history since leaving the hostel (not really at our wish) has been one of repeated prosecutions: for larceny, for assault, for taking and driving away, for breach of probation. He has been once in a detention centre, twice in psychiatric hospitals, once in borstal. He has twice attempted his own life, has had a liaison with a young wife with two children, was chronically unable to keep a job or lodgings, but was always confident that his troubles would soon be over, that now he had 'learned his lesson'. All this happened before he reached the age of twenty-one. During all this young man's diversity of tribulation close contact was maintained. He was often visited in his various places of incarceration; if we knew of them in time we attended his court hearings; when he was sick in a bedsitter, my wife acted as a kind of district nurse; he visited the hostel often, and when the residents turned against him, he visited us in our flat; and he spent his home leave with us in our house in the country. All this was because one of Eustace's chronic emotional needs was for parent substitutes, and he had cast us in that role. We cannot escape the conviction that in the particular work in which we are engaged such a demand must be granted, and once granted its continuance becomes an inescapable personal responsibility which may not be shed until the boy no longer needs it. The degree to which Eustace's misery has been alleviated by this relationship cannot be measured, and amelioration of this kind, while no substitute for healing, is a mercy not to be despised. Experience has convinced us that such a relationship, staunchly and unconditionally maintained can in the end make possible the success of other therapeutic influences which, in its absence, are almost bound to fail. This is what I wrote in my formal report about Eustace; since it was written Eustace has come out of borstal, and thanks to a devoted borstal aftercare volunteer, has had a longer period of employment and general stability than he has ever enjoyed. The last thing I want to do is to belittle the work of that devoted man and his wife. But I feel fairly confident that if we had not 'hung on' to him during all those crises and misadventures, he would have found it less possible to accept what those admirable people offer.

Of thirty-eight leavers, no fewer than ten left prematurely, seven of them in the hostel's first year. This high wastage rate at the beginning was of course due to what are commonly called teething troubles, and wastage in the remaining four years was extremely low, less than one a year. Perhaps the chief teething trouble was over-anxiety to fill the hostel, so that selection became too elastic. In spite of what I said in an earlier chapter about the conditions we laid down, several boys in the early days did not meet those requirements. Two boys had not been to schools for maladjusted children, two did not come straight from such schools, three were accepted before the psychiatrist had been appointed. It must also be said that among this group of ten premature leavers, were three about whom we had been misled by people anxious to get them into the hostel. We were given information about them which was not merely incomplete, which one could perhaps almost forgive, but which was in places simply not true.

Two of these premature leavers were expelled on account of their violence. Two others left at our request; they were found to be much too grossly disturbed, and their sponsors were asked to remove them. Of the remaining six, two absconded and did not return, three insisted for various reasons on returning to their families and one was committed to an approved school.

In spite of all these misadventures it seems probable that if some of these premature leavers had come to the hostel when it was firmly established instead of in its early days we might very well have done something for them. Their average length of stay was fourteen weeks, and we have called them 'negative leavers' because we do not profess to have done anything with them; they did not stay long enough to become well integrated into the community, they did not make affective relationships, and we distinguish them from the other 'positive' leavers, some of whom may indeed have left very early but not before they had established affective ties of one kind or another. The boy, for example, who never settled at the hostel and was so grossly disturbed that we asked his sponsors to remove him after three or four months, belongs properly to a different category from Arthur who was prepared to settle and got on well with staff and residents, but who was taken away by his father in a fit of remorse after four or five months. Another way of putting it, is to say that the boys we have described as negative leavers never really accepted the hostel or (less frequently) were not accepted by it, so that they did not remain long enough to justify being included in the general figures of outcome. Aftercare was in those cases not provided because they immediately reverted to the care of those in whose care they had hitherto been, or passed into the care of others who would thereafter be responsible for them; and because aftercare is thought of as having as an important constituent part, the continuance of an affective tie already made. With these ten negative leavers there was no such tie.

The following observations about outcome apply only to the twenty boys who are designated positive leavers because, whatever the circumstances of their leaving, a solid relationship had been built up and was continued so long as was felt necessary after the boy had left.

The average length of stay of these boys was twenty months, ranging between five months and thirty-three. All but five have at the time of writing been gone for a year or more. The average age on leaving was 17, ranging between 15 years 10 months, and 18 years 7 months.

Criteria for an assessment of outcome are difficult to establish because so many imponderable and subjective judgements are involved. No sharp dividing line can be drawn between success and failure, but if regard is taken to steadiness of employment, the number (if any) of court appearances, committals to institutions (penal or psychiatric), ability to keep lodgings, and personal appearance and manner, it is

H

found in practice that the boys who have left can be placed in six fairly clearly defined groups:

1	Exceptionally good progress	5 boys
2	Satisfactory progress	6 boys
3	Outcome so far doubtful	4 boys
4	Progress unsatisfactory	2 boys
5	Transferred to other establishments	2 boys
6	Only just left	1 boy

Total   20 boys

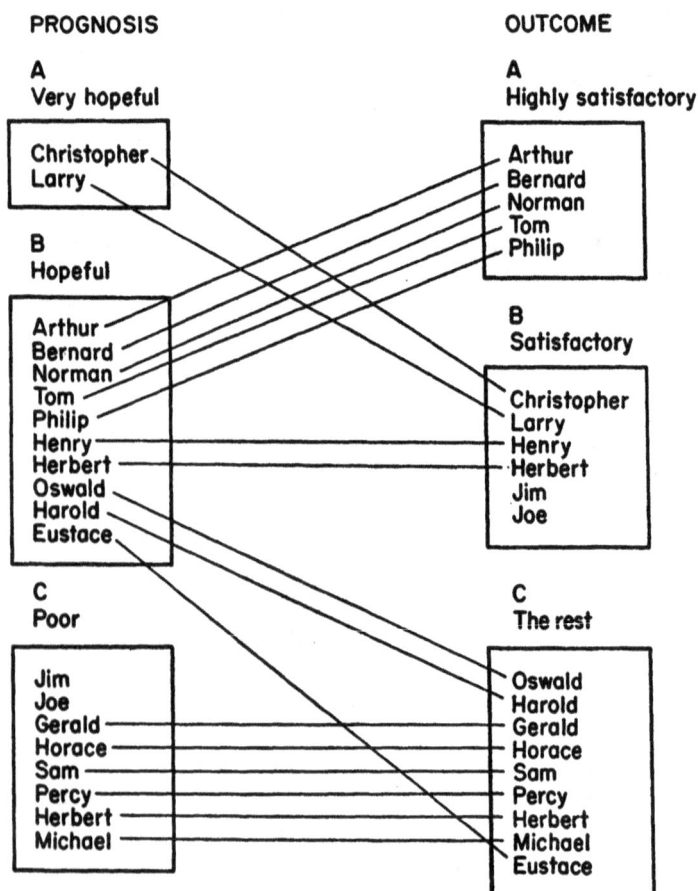

Chart to show prognosis of boys' development relative to outcome.

Although these are clearly defined groups, it will be convenient for practical purposes to collect all the last four into one group, so that we have three main groups: A, highly satisfactory; B, satisfactory, and C, the rest.

While it is difficult to make even the roughest assessment of outcome, which really cannot be judged for at least five years after discharge, even such judgement as can be made is of little use in assessing the value of the hostel's work unless it is related to our expectations. If those expectations are maintained or exceeded it may be thought that the effort and money expended have been justified. If expectations are not maintained, it may well be thought that the hostel has not justified its existence. The twenty leavers have therefore been placed in prognostic categories (which the psychiatrist and I worked out between us), based on expectations at the time of admission. Here again we made three groups, roughly equivalent to the three given above: group A, very hopeful; group B, hopeful; and Group C, poor.

Before giving the figures for these prognostic groups however, a word of explanation is called for. The likely future of a person who is emotionally disturbed will depend to a large degree on the environment (primarily the human environment) in which he finds himself. All the boys who came to Reynolds House did so because the people concerned for their future were pretty confident that in any normal environment that was available for them, the prognosis was very poor. In this sense expectations might be said to be low for all of them, and they could all be put in prognostic group C. Our judgement, however, in making these allocations was based on the assumption that they would be coming to the relatively favourable environment of Reynolds House; if we say the outlook for a given boy is good, we mean that it is good only if he is first to enjoy for a reasonable period the favourable environment of the hostel.

Even bearing this in mind, then, we did not feel that we could assign more than two boys to the 'very hopeful' category, when they arrived, and then somewhat doubtfully. But as has been said, five boys were described as 'highly satisfactory' when they left. In the 'hopeful' group B, we placed ten boys, which compares with only six satisfactory leavers; and we put eight in the C (poor prognosis) group, which compares with nine in the C outcome group. It must be borne in mind however that the C outcome includes the boy who has just left, the four described as doubtful, and the two who were transferred to full time residential treatment.

All this rather complicated grouping can perhaps best be displayed in a chart in which it is possible to see what has happened to each boy. From this it will be clear that the two doubtful A prognoses did not in fact fulfil expectation, though their outcome is still satisfactory. On the other hand, five B prognoses achieved an A outcome, while two maintained their status. Of the three B prognoses whose outcome was designated C, one is the recent leaver, one is still doubtful, and only one is a clear descent from B to C.

Of the eight C prognoses, there were two promotions to B outcomes, leaving six in this group of whom the worst that can be said of them is that they did no better than was expected of them, but even so, only one is at this stage clearly to be seen as unsatisfactory.

CHAPTER TEN

AN UNSUCCESSFUL ATTEMPT AT EVALUATION

Evaluation of a piece of work of this kind is in any circumstances very difficult. That difficulty is enhanced when the project is near in time to evaluation, and its objectivity is open to serious question when it is being made by people who were responsible for carrying out the work. Nevertheless, certain questions can be asked, and an effort made to give tentative replies to them. It is also possible to make a few general observations.

To deal first with the questions:

1 Is the demand for such hostels as great as had been assumed?

On this our experience at Reynolds House provides at best only the most inconclusive evidence because we had great difficulty in keeping the hostel full. This astonished me because I knew from my own experience as head of a school for maladjusted children, as well as from my conversations with fellow heads, that there is a very great need for some such facility, and I expected that we should be inundated with applications. Yet, in spite of what I should have thought was more than adequate publicity, it was eighteen months before the hostel was full. As this question is a crucial one, it would be well to look a little further into it. There appear to be two reasons to account for the effective demand being less than we anticipated. The first emerged when the hostel had been running for about eighteen months, and para-doxically it seemed to be the very size of the problem that led to our being inadequately used. Our unfilled state caused me such surprise and concern that I frequently referred to it in conversation with friends and colleagues in the work, and more than one of them replied that as we had only twelve beds and there was such a great demand for such a hostel, school authorities and social workers with a boy to place would take it for granted that we should be full and would not even bother to apply. This seemed such a far-fetched theory that for some time I ignored it, but at length I heard it so often that I acted on it. In the spring of 1965, eighteen months after opening, there were still only eight boys in residence, and no applications in sight, so I wrote to a few headmasters of my acquaintance saying it was not true that we were full up, and if they had a boy for whom our services might be useful, they would do well to let us know. That summer's school-leavers produced more applicants than we could deal with, so that for some months there were thirteen boys in the hostel. From that time onwards we adopted the regular practice of informing a few schools whenever any vacancies were imminent, and by this means kept the hostel full. When our retirement began to loom on the horizon this practice was dropped, as it was not thought desirable to receive new boys just before we left, and applications dropped off. Far-fetched as it seemed therefore, there evidently was something in the suggestion that people did not bother to enquire because they felt so sure we should be full up.

The second reason for the lack of urgency in demand may seem speculative, but seems to me quite probable. It may be said to be due to a kind of administrative gap which appears just at the point when a boy is leaving school and the need for a placement of this kind appears. The people who are most likely to be acutely conscious of the need for a particular boy are those at his school, or the clinic which first referred him to the school. But the school has no statutory respon-sibility for aftercare, and neither of course has the clinic. If that responsibility rests clearly on the shoulders of any public authority, it is the mental health department; but though several applications were made by such authorities, none ever actually initiated one. They were initiated by schools or clinics, who then persuaded the medical officer of health to make the formal application. Of thirty-eight accepted applications, no fewer than twenty-four were initiated by schools, four by child guidance clinics, nine by children's departments and one by a youth employment officer. This is more remarkable than it might seem at first sight. It is true that the headmaster is more likely than anyone to be aware of the boy's needs, but it is also true that he has no further responsibility for a boy once he leaves school, and might well be forgiven for assuming that the proper care of the boy is now someone else's business. In spite of this, however, two-thirds of the boys who came to us did so at the instance of their schools, and this is even more remarkable when we examine the difficulties which con-front a headmaster who seeks a hostel placement. First he has to discover a suitable hostel, when there are altogether only four hostels for maladjusted school-leavers in existence and three of them are primarily for boys from specific schools. Then he has to discover the procedure for admission, and what statutory authorities, if any, are empowered to bear the cost of such a placement. Then he not only has to persuade them to pay in this particular case, sometimes he even has to convince them that they do indeed have the power to do so.

If the boy should happily chance to be already in care, the difficulties are not so great, because the school will already have been in touch with the child care officer (though of course the school's primary responsibility for the boy has always been to the education authority), and the children's department already has financial responsibility for the boy. The child care officer has probably been wondering what he will do with the boy when he leaves school, and is only too delighted to act on any good suggestion the school may make. But only a small proportion of the boys in schools for maladjusted children are in care, and for the others the position is very different. It must be remembered also not only that all this is very time-consuming for the headmaster, and it is consuming time in a field which is technically not his responsibility, but he is now moving in an area with which he is usually quite unfamiliar, and in which, apart from a few exceptional cases, he does not have any expertise. That a headmaster should be familiar with the education acts and the work of education authorities we may well expect; that he should be equally familiar with the mental health acts and the work of mental health departments is more than we are entitled to suppose. It may be relatively easy for a person of authority and wide-ranging experience, for example, like the late head of the Caldecott Community, to surmount all these difficulties, as she did in three cases. But one cannot be surprised if more ordinary mortals find it all too daunting and let it drop. After all, it is not their responsibility, nor that of their employers.

In short, at the very point at which the need arises, responsibility is passed – by those who are most conscious of the need – to an entirely different set of people, or none, who have never before heard of the boy in question and who need to be convinced, if anyone feels strongly enough about it to do so, of the need, which even then of course they will not feel as strongly about as those who have had the care of the boy in all the preceding years.

One cannot forbear to express the view that if the aftercare service, including hostels, were to rest with the Department of Education and Science (and thus with local education authorities), this problem would disappear. The concerned headmaster would then merely have to telephone a familiar figure at his education office to put the matter in train. I am certain that if that were the position, the effective demand for places would be such as to set up a great demand for more hostels. In this connection it is interesting to note that of the twenty-four applications initiated by schools, only three were not initiated by people who were already sufficiently familiar with me to be able easily to telephone, as did the redoubtable head of the Caldecott Community and say 'How do I set about getting a boy into your hostel?' And three of the four clinic applications started in the same way.

The next question that might be asked is:

2 Did the boys presented for admission prove to be of the kind that had been expected?

Of the kind, yes; but bearing in mind the requirement of the selection criteria that the boy was expected to have made some progress towards stability, the degree of the problems presented was more serious than we had anticipated. It will have become clear that the boys who came to the hostel were still quite seriously disturbed people for whom it was necessary to provide not only a stable home background but also a good deal of skilled therapeutic support. Without this there is very little doubt that most of them would have failed.

The third question is:

3 Did the staffing prove to be adequate and appropriate?

In the main, yes. The point made in (2) above caused greater demands on the psychiatrist than had been bargained for as more boys were in need of psychotherapy than had been considered likely. Before the end of the five-year period it had become clear to the staff that it would have been a great help if the psychiatrist had had time for at least a few psychotherapeutic interviews. It was thought that this might very well have affected outcome favourably in several cases, either by reducing the amount of time the boy needed to stay in the hostel or (more often) by achieving a greater degree of stability. There were nine boys of whom it was thought that they might have been much helped by psychotherapy, but the idea of going to a clinic or hospital for outpatient treatment would have been (in one or two cases was demonstrated to be) quite unacceptable to them. They would, however, undoubtedly have accepted it as it were at home, from a person they already knew and liked, and it seems a great pity that established relationships could not have been capitalized in this way. It may not be true to say of psychotherapy that the establishment of a good rapport with the patient is half the battle, but it is certainly an essential prerequisite, and here it was already to hand, but, for this purpose at least, unutilized. It might have been feasible to ask the psychiatrist to come weekly instead of fortnightly, and, by holding the case conference monthly instead of fortnightly, to release him for at least six consultations a month. This proposition was not put forward during the period of office of our first psychiatrist because she would probably not have been able to give us the time anyway. By the time her successor arrived I was more or less on my way out, and it was thought better to hold this matter in abeyance until my successor was in post. So the proposition was never formally put forward.

On the other hand, there were at first fewer demands on the psychiatric social worker than had been anticipated, because of the total and irremediable breach between most of the boys and their families. But for the same reason aftercare became more important than had originally been envisaged.

It may also be said that my wife's preoccupation with domestic chores prevented her from making the fullest use of her particular gifts and expertise in the therapeutic field, and that this problem might have been solved by spending more on daily domestics. But in domestic work, even more than in many others, Parkinson's Law is an ever present danger. And, as has been said, the very fact that the womenfolk were so often engaged in domestic work made them more readily accessible to the boys, and much of therapeutic value might have been lost if they had not been so occupied, hard though it was on them.

4 Are the methods employed at Reynolds House capable of general application in any future hostels?

What I have written here hardly provides any evidence on this point except insofar as I have described the methods. Methods are very important, but men are not less so, and people with a concern for the work and with a suitable background of training and experience might have equal or greater success using methods quite different from those described here. Again, nothing that has been written here provides any evidence as to whether people who are capable of using successfully these or any other methods are to be found. That they are not easily to be found I am sure. Residential work of any kind appeals to very few people, and hostel work as I found to my great surprise is more trying than most. A high degree of skill and training is called for, but the scale of pay in hostel work in general is still far below that of the teaching profession for example. And teachers consider themselves a grossly underpaid profession. Insofar as such people are to be found, the probability is that this is more likely in the field of the education of the maladjusted than in the general field of residential child care because their experience and training is likely to be more closely related to the problems presented by maladjusted children. For them however such a move would probably involve a considerable drop in pay.

5 Would there have been much advantage in having girls as well as boys in the hostel?

In my view, no. I am a firm believer in co-education, for the usual kind of reasons, but in the particular circumstances of Reynolds House the disadvantages of a one-sex establishment are so minimal that the administrative difficulties of a mixed hostel outweighed them. This is not to say that I am opposed to mixed hostels, but merely that it does not very much matter whether they are mixed or not. In the hostel situation there is ample opportunity for boys and girls to meet each other, at work and at play, and having met they can bring their boy- or girl-friends 'home'. There are far more boys than girls in schools for maladjusted children, so if there are to be many more hostels the majority of them will have to be boys' hostels. I will not go into all the little administrative difficulties, but one of them is that unless all the residents have single rooms, the ratio of the sexes has to remain constant, and it might well happen that when there is a girl's vacancy all the applicants are boys, and vice versa. This means that there is liable to be an empty bed or beds for no other reason than that the hostel is a mixed one, and this is financially disastrous in a small hostel.

My experience of running a small mixed hostel (which I did for a short time) does not lead me to expect what is commonly called 'trouble between the boys and girls'. The residents tend to be much of an age, and as boys want younger girls and girls seek older boys, they all tend to seek their friends of the opposite sex outside the hostel.

6 Can the hostel be said to have justified its existence looked at both socially and financially?

(a) The boys admitted to Reynolds House were by definition those who in the opinion of their sponsors were going to break down if on leaving school they went to any other available kind of accommodation. Fifteen out of the twenty boys have not so far broken down in this way, so fifteen expected breakdowns have been averted. This seems ample justification socially.

(b) It is not so easy to make a judgement of this kind on financial grounds. This is partly because there are many ways of counting the financial cost. I can make one calculation which will make it appear that each of these averted breakdowns cost society £4,000. I can make another that puts it at £3,000, and I can make still a third from which it appears that the money actually spent on each satisfactory leaver was about £1,000. It is not very important how I arrive at these different figures. Whether the expense of £1,000 a head, or £4,000 a head is justified, is not a financial question, but a moral and political one, as there is no means by which a price can be put upon a human life saved from mental and social breakdown. It can fairly safely be said, however, that, given the original premise that these were all potential breakdowns, much more than £4,000 would have been spent by society on each of these boys if the expected breakdowns had indeed taken place.

7 By whom should any further hostels be set up and administered? This is another question on which our experience is not such as to supply a complete answer. Reynolds House was set up and administered by a voluntary body, as also were the three other hostels known to me: Easton House, The Gatehouse, and the hostel run by Bodenham Manor School. For us this was a happy and satisfactory arrangement, except in one particular to which I shall refer; but if there are to be many more hostels of this kind it is hardly to be expected that the money for all of them will come from voluntary sources. The question then arises which government department or which department of the local authority should be responsible for such a service?

The Underwood Committee seemed to have little doubt that it should be placed securely in the lap of the local education authority. This is perhaps not the place to go into all the pros and cons of such a recommendation, but our experience at Reynolds House does reveal one factor strongly in its support, namely, that a service so administered is much more likely to be fully used, and the occupancy was the one particular just mentioned in which our administrative arrangements seemed to fall short. If the other existing hostels have not experienced this difficulty to the same degree, this may well be because they were established primarily to meet the needs of a specific school. There is much to be said for this, though the probability is that no one school (unless it were a very large one, and no school for maladjusted children should be very large) is likely to have a sufficient number of suitable leavers to keep a hostel full. A consortium of schools jointly running a hostel might be more practicable, but even then only if public funds were available.

I write however at a time when the recommendations of the Seebohm Committee are being incorporated in a bill to unify the administration of the social services, and if the bill is enacted, modifications will clearly be necessary in what I have just said. Presumably in such a case the appropriate body to accept responsibility for hostels of many kinds, including hostels for maladjusted school-leavers, would be the social services department of the local authority. This would certainly solve the problem of the headmaster wondering which department to approach in seeking a placement for a boy. It would also, it seems to me, have a further and far-reaching effect. If the social services are really integrated, and if the Children and Young Persons Act of 1969 really succeeds in its plan to incorporate what were once approved schools into a system of community homes, a further development becomes possible. There are many young people with the same kind of background, the same problems and the same general needs as those leaving schools for maladjusted children. A unified, integrated social service would be able to establish hostels for such youngsters irrespective of their immediate provenance, and this would be a great gain. Within this service different hostels could have different emphases and deal with different specific needs and degrees of need in much the same way as in the proposed community homes. This again would be a great gain, though I do see one serious danger in it. The child moving from an earlier placement to an after-care hostel often needs for some time to maintain affective ties built up in the establishment from which he is moving, and it seems to me that this rationalization of hostel services would make that more difficult. For that purpose the ideal arrangement would seem to be for schools to run their own hostels, jointly or collectively as I suggested above. But perhaps that is an impossible ideal; it is certainly at variance in an administrative sense to anything that is likely in the present Bill.

There is one more thing I must say, though it is not strictly relevant to the work of the hostel, but our experience there did highlight a need for which there is virtually no provision. This relates to the many applications made on behalf of maladjusted boys who failed to qualify for admission because they had never been at a school for maladjusted children. Whether a hostel is the appropriate placement for all these boys I very much doubt. Certainly a number of them have needs that a hostel can hardly be expected to supply. One feels that for some of them the solution might be found in a residential establishment which purports to do for the adolescent what the school attempts to do for the child. That is to say, the establishment would be work-oriented, as the school is, except that the work would be in field, garden or workshop instead of the classroom; and the treatment would be, as the school's is, a form of environmental therapy based on and working through affective relationships. Whether this type of regime would be more effective than the clinical type of therapy provided by hospitals I am not concerned at the moment to discuss; what is quite certain is that it would be immeasurably more acceptable to the subject, and would militate against the danger of his thinking of himself as a sick person, or as an 'interesting case'.

So I find myself, at the end of my working life still pleading for the kind of establishment which I tried to demonstrate in use at the beginning of it.[1] At any rate, the climate now is much more favourable than it was then, so perhaps there is at last some hope.

[1] See the *Hawkspur Experiment*, by W. David Wills, George Allen & Unwin, London, 1968.

INDEX

For Product Safety Concerns and Information please contact our EU
representative GPSR@taylorandfrancis.com
Taylor & Francis Verlag GmbH, Kaufingerstraße 24, 80331 München, Germany

www.ingramcontent.com/pod-product-compliance
Lightning Source LLC
Chambersburg PA
CBHW050523280326
41932CB00014B/2436

9 781032 067346